PLANI
BASED
DIET
MANUAL

Proven Strategies To Lose Weight &
Gain Muscle On A Plant Based Diet

M.G. Green

www.amazon.com/author/mggreen

fiveminutediet@gmail.com

@fiveminutediet (Instagram)

ISBN-13: 978-1974468423

ISBN-10: 1974468429

Table Of Contents

Intro

One of the most common issues among Vegans is the ability to obtain a lean and chiseled physique. Now, this statement goes completely against the "skinny vegan" stereotype, however this is the reality faced by many who adhere to a plant-based diet.

The decision to not consume animal products leaves Vegans with even less lean sources of protein to choose from. This can lead to overeating "not as lean" foods and eventually cause body-fat.

Despite this, there are still scores of individuals that thrive on a strict, plant-based regimen. The difference between these individuals and those who struggle is very simple. Those that thrive:

1. made the decision to invest in nutritional knowledge
2. have a high level of self-control with food choices
3. prepare and/or cook for themselves consistently
4. are active and participate in some sort of physical exercise
5. have and follow an actual plan to reach specific goals

This book addresses all of these concepts. I want you to view these concepts as skills. The more you improve at each skill, the better you will look and feel. I cannot state this any clearer!

I cover two forms of Vegan dieting in this book. The first is traditional whole food, plant-based eating. I go over the foods, the macro-nutrient counts, the calories-counts—*everything* you need to know to accomplish specific goals on this type of diet.

The second form is aimed at those with extremely busy lifestyles. Taste, time, convenience, and on-the-go eating are prioritized without sacrificing results. To the point where I have tested using only five-minute meals (over multiple week stretches), and still simultaneously gained muscle and lost body-fat.

I want you to treat this book as a **guide**. Look over the Food Lists. Follow the instructions and implement the strategies. It's a quick read as each section is straight to the point. This guide is designed to be reusable and easily referenced.

Saying this, feel free to skip around the chapters. Go straight to the topic that catches your eye and begin from there! The time is now to take control of your health and body!

1 What To Eat

Eating so-called "clean" is not difficult. It truly isn't—I promise you this. There are several reasons why we fail to take complete control of our nutrition on a consistent basis, but let's first address the solutions.

The reality is this:

It is 21st Century. If you are fortunate enough to live in the "civilized world", you have complete control over what you *choose* to eat and drink. Recognizing this, let me throw at you a starter list of healthy food options. This will be an incomplete list—it will not contain every single healthy (clean) food possible! The list will serve as a reference when: grocery shopping, cooking, and eating out.

We will not focus just yet on how certain foods can or should be prepared—Chapter 3 will cover this.

Food List

The Food List will be split into 5 categories: **Proteins**, **Carbohydrates**, **Fats**, **Vegetables**, and **Fruit**. These categorizations are put in place to make "meal building" (Chapter 3) extremely simple. Keep in mind that many whole foods are versatile and can dip into multiple categories.

For example:

- I list several types of beans under carbohydrates. Beans are also a good source of protein. However, they are not (generally) considered a lean protein. Beans contain significant calories from *both* complex carbohydrates, and protein.
- All fruits and vegetables are forms of carbohydrates. Keep in mind that not all carbohydrates are created equally.
- Nuts and seeds are generally considered "fats". They do, however, also contain both carbohydrates and protein.
- While leafy greens are considered vegetables, they are also relatively high in protein (~1g/10 calories on average)

Food List

Look over the the food list. Make note of any foods you enjoy, or want to try.

Proteins

Plant Protein Powder (pg. 55-57)
Tofu
Tempeh (from soybeans)*

*Tempeh is fermented. Keep track of how it affects your body (digestion, energy, skin, etc). I do not eat tempeh. I much prefer tofu due to the taste, texture, leanness, and lack of fermentation. As you will read later on, this diet plan does not include fermented foods, yeast, probiotics, and the like. Obviously you can bend the rules if you prefer to. The same goes with "seitan" aka vital wheat gluten ("fake" meat).

Fats

Peanuts / Peanut Butter
Almonds / Almond Butter
Cashews / Cashew Butter
Hazelnuts / Hazelnut Butter
Pistachios
Brazil Nuts
Chestnuts
Macadamia Nuts
Pecans
Pine Nuts
Walnuts
Extra Virgin Coconut Oil
Extra Virgin Olive Oil
Canola Oil
Safflower Oil
Sunflower Oil
Hemp Seeds
Chia Seeds
Pumpkin Seeds
Sesame Seeds / Tahini
Sunflower Seeds / Butter / Oil
Flax Seeds / Oil
Avocados
Cacao / Cacao Butter
Dark Chocolate (80% or higher)

Carbohydrates

Brown Rice
Wild Rice
Buckwheat
Rolled Oats (Gluten-Free)
Quinoa
Aramanth
Millet
Corn

Lentils
Garbanzo Beans (Chickpeas)
Kidney Beans
Black Beans
Soy Beans/Edamame
Cannelloni Beans
Mung Beans
Lima Beans
Green Beans
Adzuki Beans
Peas

Sweet Potatoes
Yams

Vegetables

Broccoli
Kale
Spinach
Romaine Lettuce
Arugula
Okra
Cabbage
Brussels Sprouts
Carrots
Cauliflower
Beets
Mushrooms*
Eggplant
Zucchini
Squash
Yellow Onions
White Onions
Green Onions (Scallions)
Leeks
Red Onions
Red Peppers
Green Peppers
Yellow Peppers
Orange Peppers
Celery
Cucumbers

*I do not eat mushrooms. This isn't to say one shouldn't, but track how they affect your digestion.

Fruits

Tomatoes
Strawberries
Blueberries
Blackberries
Raspberries
Mango
Pineapple
Papaya
Cantaloupe
Melon
Watermelon
Peaches
Banana
Apples
Pears
Oranges
Tangerines
Grapes
Cherries
Lemons
Limes
Kiwis
Apricots
Figs

Spices

Here is a beginner list of spices. Spices can be added to foods in abundance. Do not worry about limiting them! Learning how to use and combine spices is very important. Taste is *vital* for long-term compliance.

Black Pepper	Cinnamon
Garlic / Garlic Powder	Cayenne Pepper
Onion Powder	Cloves
Basil	Ginger
Oregano	Fennel
Parsley	Thyme
Turmeric	Parsley
Cumin	Saffron
Chili	Rosemary
Paprika	Cilantro

Salt

You can have salt, but do not abuse it. Feel free to sprinkle lightly on meals every once in a while. Keep in mind that many nut butters contain salt (peanut butter, almond butter, etc)—even the healthy ones. If you are a person who loves salted peanut butter (for example), perhaps it would be a good idea to lay off adding salt to your stir-fries. There are also nut butters that do not contain salt (these are what I use). They taste just as good.

Again, consume in moderation and feel free to experiment with the several forms: Sea Salt, Himalayan Salt, Regular Salt, etc. Salt is similar to sugar in that: the less you eat it, the less you will crave it.

Protein

I want to address a few topics in regards to plant-based protein.

Lean Protein

If you were to look at the "Nutrition Facts" label of a food deemed a "lean protein", you would see (per serving) a high amount of protein (~10-20g+), an extremely low amount of carbs (~0g), and a relatively low amount of fat (a few grams tops).

The ideology of lean protein sources is that the majority of calories come from just protein, and therefore will not be a potential cause of (an increase in) body-fat. This is actually true, but it does not mean that "non-lean sources" (beans, for example) *will* cause body-fat. Body-fat is primarily caused by eating unhealthy foods or simply too much food. Not to mention: failing to exercise (sedentary lifestyles).

Complete Proteins

Most plant-based protein sources are not considered "complete" sources of protein (soybeans are an exception). A complete protein contains all nine essential amino acids in the proper proportions (amounts). Amino acids are the building blocks of protein.

There are both essential and non-essential amino acids:
- Essential amino acids are not produced by our bodies. Therefore, it is "essential" that we consume them.
- Non-essential amino acids are already produced (synthesized) by our bodies. It is not essential that we consume them.

The necessity of consuming a complete protein at every meal is always a hot topic of debate. Do we really *need* all nine essential amino acids in the proper amounts each and every meal?

 Side 1: "No. As long as we eat a variety of plant-based whole foods throughout the day, our bodies will absorb sufficient amounts of each of the nine essential amino acids."

 Side 2: "Of course we do! Each meal is a new meal. Our body hungers to be refueled. The fuel should be **optimized** *to the max*. More amino acids is better than less amino acids."

What is my take on this?

The competitor in me naturally leans toward "Side 2" ... but then I see relatively in-shape Vegans claim "Side 1" ... but then I see those same "Side 1" people supplementing with protein powder and claiming it is strictly for taste!

My conclusion: try for "Side 2" as much as possible, but it isn't the end of the world if a meal (or snack) leans towards "Side 1". Beans can absolutely serve as a primary source of protein. Not only for a meal or two, but for the majority of a person's diet. I will provide examples of this in Chapter 3.

Fats

The term "fats" is not to be confused with body-fat. Fats are one of the three macro-nutrients that make up foods (in addition to protein and carbohydrates). Consuming fats does not equate to gaining body-fat. Companies try to use this potential confusion as a marketing tactic. "Low-fat", "reduced fat", "zero fat" – this is all garbage and should be disregarded. In fact, if you see one of these labels, run the other way. It often means that the (healthy) fat portion was removed, and replaced with either some sort of chemical or sweetener.

Saying this, fats *do happen* to be extremely caloric. This, however, is not a reason to avoid them. It is simply a reason to *physically* measure your intake per meal.

Carbohydrates ("carbs")

As I mentioned earlier, there are several forms of carbohydrates. To keep things simple, we will look at three potential categorizations: simple carbs (aka simple sugars), complex carbs (aka starches), and dietary fiber. We will first discuss simple carbs and complex carbs.

The primary difference between simple carbs and complex carbs (other than chemical structure) is how the body processes each. Simple carbs raise blood sugar (glucose) levels far quicker than complex carbs. Simple carbs are also not reliable sources for long-term energy.

An example of a simple carbohydrate is fructose. Fructose is found in both fruits and vegetables. The amount of fructose in these foods can vary greatly. For example: broccoli contains a small amount of fructose, while a banana contains quite a bit. Therefore, a banana will have a large effect on raising blood sugar levels—broccoli will not.

Broccoli also contains a small amount of complex carbohydrates, though it is primarily made up of fiber (similar to other vegetables). A better example of a complex carb is brown rice. Complex carbs are very reliable forms of long-term energy for the body. Complex carbs are broken down far slower than simple carbs. Generally speaking, when an individual refers to "carbs", he or she is referring to complex carbs.

As I mentioned earlier, dietary fiber is another form of carbohydrate. However, it is indigestible and not a reliable form of long-term energy. Fiber assists in the digestion of other foods.

The amount and type of simple carbs (sugars), complex carbs (starches), and dietary fiber per food item is the basis of the food categorizations:

- "carbs",
- fruits,
- and vegetables.

It isn't necessary to go into more detail here, so I won't. If you are interested in the nutritional makeup of a food item, do an internet search "<name of food> nutrition". There are sites that provide everything from standard nutritional facts (calories, protein, carbs, etc) to even amino-acid profiles. I recommend doing this when meal-building during Chapter 3.

What To Drink
Water
By far, the number one liquid you should consume is water. There are several reasons for this:

- 0 calories
- cleans out your system better than anything
- ideal for hydration

I am not going to spend much time here. This is mostly common knowledge. What I will say is: you need to drink a fair amount throughout the day. The vast majority of the population is dehydrated. Whatever amount you are drinking now, drink more. The first thing you should put in your body every morning is water (at least a glass, or bottle—immediately!). Then drink a glass or bottle with your breakfast. Then have water available for the span between meal 1 and meal 2. Then drink one during meal 2. Etc, etc, etc.

If you occasionally want some flavor, perhaps purchase one of those electrolyte/stevia-based flavored supplements to mix into your water.

Coffee & Tea
If you choose to consume coffee or tea, keep in mind that the sweetener (or creamer) is probably not compliant to this diet. Adding a legitimate sweetener (sugar, agave, etc) to one of these drinks will also do your taste-buds a massive disservice. What I mean by this is, the more you consume sweet foods or beverages, the more you will crave sweet foods and beverages. Doing this first thing in the morning is not the smartest idea in the world.

Milk Alternatives
Almond milk, cashew milk, coconut milk, soy milk, rice milk, among others. Get the unsweetened version. This can be used as a coffee creamer or in recipes (smoothies, etc). Keep in mind that these *do* have calories. When I use one of these options, I dilute it with water.

Organic vs. Non-Organic

In the plant-based world, organic refers to zero pesticides, hormones, or GMOs (genetically modified organisms). I will keep this extremely short. My advice is this: when possible and plausible (price, etc), choose organic. Saying this, eating organic can be expensive—so I am not going to say you must eat organic. Most of what I eat is not organic.

If it isn't labeled "organic" or "non-gmo", pesticides, hormones, or GMOs were used to create/cultivate it. It is that simple. These labels are a selling point. There is no reason a company would choose to not use these labels (if they could).

The vast majority of food in the "western world" does not contain one of these labels!

2 What *Not* To Eat

Now that you have an idea on what you can/should be eating, let's look at what you should not be eating. When it comes to lowering body-fat, and maintaining a low body-fat %, **the ingredients that you do not consume, are more important than the ingredients you do consume.** What I mean by this is: it is more important to avoid certain ingredients, than to make sure you "get" certain ingredients in your body.

For example: you can literally eat *just* brown rice and protein powder and attain a relatively impressive physique. Not the most nutritious diet by any means—I am referring strictly to body-fat and muscle. This will not hold true for a more well-rounded diet that also contains culprit ingredients (such as sugar and yeast).

"Calories in, calories out" is *complete* "BS" when it comes to body-fat. It aggravates me when I hear this. If "calories in vs calories out" really held true, all it would take is a caloric deficit (eating less calories than you consume) to get "ripped", "cut", "toned" – however you want to say it.

"Calories in, calories out" *may* have a short term effect in terms of the numbers on the scale. However, the numbers on the scale do not tell the whole story—not even remotely close. Dehydration techniques alone can cause a *TWENTY POUND (plus)* "weight loss" in a matter of a few days. Let this sink in. Not to mention the fact that muscle and body-fat both contribute to overall body weight.

Ingredients To Avoid

Animal Products
This diet plan is Vegan. Vegan refers to a 100% plant-based lifestyle. This includes absolutely zero ingredients that come from an animal: the flesh, bones, muscles, and organs … the milk and eggs as well.

Honey is also not Vegan. I will go over the reason(s) when I address sugars and sweeteners in the following section.

I personally chose to cut out animal products for moral reasons. It was not until weeks to months in that I realized the physical benefits. And I am not referring to the studies that potentially link animal products to diseases such as cancer and heart disease. I mean *literally* how I looked and felt. My body-fat decreased and my energy level increased. Most notably, my digestion and bowel movements completely normalized.

I will be completely honest with you: dairy is worse for humans than meat. Less immoral if they had to be compared, but definitely worse for the actual body. *All things being equal*, meat eaters that do not consume dairy are healthier than vegetarians that do consume dairy. Our digestive system does not handle dairy well. I hate to type this, but it handles cooked meat far better—especially if we are comparing it to casein.

The only form of dairy humans do not have much of an issue with is whey. A cow's milk is made up of two proteins: whey and casein. The vast majority of the protein in milk is casein—80% of it to be (more) exact. The other 20% is Whey. Casein is a **terror** on human digestive systems. So much in that supplement companies slickly spun this fact into a "benefit" to help market it. They boast its "slow digesting" properties and convince individuals that this is "better" before bed as the protein will "be in your system longer".

Think about this for a minute. "Slow digesting" being a benefit. How backwards is this? It does not take a rocket scientist to realize that slow digesting equates to "difficult to digest". Your system needs to work even harder to get this stuff through. Does it all even get through? What does it leave behind?

It shouldn't come as a surprise when I also tell you that there are studies that link casein to cancer. There are entire books devoted to the subject. If you aren't convinced of casein's unhealthiness, take the time to test it. Conjure up the discipline to go two weeks without it (assuming you are a vegetarian or still consume animal products). Cheese, yogurt, milk—essentially cut out all dairy except for whey protein powder.

Take notice of your body. All things being equal, you will have less body-fat. You will have far less stomach aches/issues. Your bowel movements will become more "normal" and regular. Your inflammation will decrease. This isn't a theory—massive amounts of people (including myself) have experienced and reported this.

I haven't even mentioned the hormones and antibiotics found in both dairy and meat. Sketchy beyond belief. I can't help but laugh when I hear individuals (that consume dairy) make the claim that soy leads to an estrogen increase. A myth they read about versus their own reality. Soy contains "phytoestrogens" aka plant estrogen, not the human hormone "estrogen". There is zero evidence that phyto-estrogen has an effect on human estrogen levels. And to be completely honest, the industry that wants people to believe this in the first place, is the same industry that tortures and murders innocent animals by the *billions*.

In regards to meat … I am of the opinion that the "meat is not healthy" angle is extremely ineffective. There are far too many healthy individuals out there that consume *massive* amounts of meat. Individuals that live to be 100. Individuals that run a sub-5-minute mile. Individuals whose blood panels are completely normal. Not eating meat needs to be made about morality and murder. The decision to purchase meat, plus the concept of supply and demand, equates to murder. There is no other way to slice it. These animals do not die of natural causes by the billions. They are murdered.

Sugar
On a lighter note, let's talk sugar. There are various forms of sugar— I am not going to mention them all. Just know that they vary in degrees of "unhealthiness". I want to address the ones you see on nutrition labels. Before we get into specific types, know that the amount of sugar being consumed also needs to be taken into consideration. Is the sugar-type near the beginning of the ingredient list, or the end? If it is near the beginning, be assured that the product is basically "all sugar". If it is near the end, there is (generally speaking) less sugar than the former. This still does not mean the product is healthy! Check the amount of sugars and carbohydrates on the nutrition facts label. (Side note: One gram of sugar also equates to one gram of carbohydrates.)

Forms of Sugar

Sweetener	Type	Glycemic Index (approx.)
Maltodextrin	Sugar	110
Maltose	Sugar	105
Dextrose	Sugar	100
Glucose	Sugar	100
Trehalose	Sugar	70
High Fructose Corn Syrup-42	Modified Sugar	68
Sucrose	Sugar	65
Caramel	Modified Sugar	60
Golden Syrup	Modified Sugar	60
Inverted Sugar	Modified Sugar	60
Refiners Syrup	Modified Sugar	60
High Fructose Corn Syrup-55	Modified Sugar	58
Blackstrap Molasses	Sugar Extract	55
Maple Syrup	Natural Sugar	54
Honey (not Vegan)	Natural Sugar	50
Sorghum Syrup	Natural Sugar	50
Lactose (not Vegan)	Sugar	45
Cane Juice	Sugar Extract	43
Barley Malt Syrup	Modified Sugar	42
Hydrogenated Starch Hydrosylates	Sugar Alcohol	35
Coconut Palm Sugar	Natural Sugar	35
Maltitol	Sugar Alcohol	35
High Fructose Corn Syrup-90	Modified Sugar	31
Brown Rice Syrup	Modified Sugar	25
Fructose	Sugar	25
Galactose	Sugar	25

Agave Syrup	Modified Sugar	15
Xylitol	Sugar Alcohol	12
Glycerol	Sugar Alcohol	5
Sorbitol	Sugar Alcohol	4
Lactitol	Sugar Alcohol	3
Isomalt	Sugar Alcohol	2
Mannitol	Sugar Alcohol	2
Erythritol	Sugar Alcohol	1
Yacon Syrup	Natural Sweetener	1
Oligofructose	Sugar Fiber	1
Inulin	Sugar Fiber	1
Brazzein	Natural Sweetener	0
Curculin	Natural Sweetener	0
Glycyrrhizin	Natural Sweetener	0
Luo Han Guo	Natural Sweetener	0
Miraculin	Natural Sweetener	0
Monellin	Natural Sweetener	0
Pentadin	Natural Sweetener	0
Stevia	Natural Sweetener	0
Thaumatin	Natural Sweetener	0
Acesulfame K	Artificial Sweetener	0
Alitame	Artificial Sweetener	0
Aspartame	Artificial Sweetener	0
Cyclamate	Artificial Sweetener	0
Neotame	Artificial Sweetener	0
Saccharin	Artificial Sweetener	0
Sucralose	Artificial Sweetener	0

Source: "Glycemic Index for Sweeteners." *Sugar and Sweetener Guide*. N.p., n.d. Web. 6 June 2017. <http://www.sugar-and-sweetener-guide.com/glycemic-index-for-sweeteners.html>.

Glycemic Index refers to how much these forms of sugar will raise an individual's blood sugar levels. This is extremely important for diabetics. Diabetics must monitor and control blood sugar levels throughout the day. All carbohydrates have an effect on blood sugar levels—not just sweeteners.

However, glycemic index does not account for portion sizes. Another term, **glycemic load**, is calculated off of glycemic index and brings portion size into consideration.

Glycemic Load = (Glycemic Index **X** Carbs per serving) / 100

Food Item	Serving Size	Glyc. Index	Glyc. Load
White Potato	150g | 30g carb	85	26 (high | >20)
Banana	120g | 25g carb	51	13 (avg. | 10-20)
Strawberries	120g | 3g carb	40	1 (low | <10)

Keep in mind that **all** highly processed sugars can lead to what is known as "insulin resistance" (cells fail to respond normally to the hormone insulin). This includes processed forms of fructose that are otherwise "low glycemic" (e.g., agave nectar and fructose itself isolated from the fruit and listed as an ingredient).

These ingredients should be consumed sparingly and/or in small amounts. Traditional white sugar, high fructose corn syrup, and the like should be avoided altogether. In reality, they should *all* be avoided (except fruits and veggies). However, some are obviously worse than others.

Coconut sugar is a natural, lower-glycemic alternative that does a decent job at mocking the taste of traditional sugar. Keep in mind that it still is not healthy as it primarily consists of sugar. Anything that mocks the taste of sugar "too well" also contains sugar!

An even better alternative is stevia. Stevia does not mock the taste of traditional sugar all that well. However if used properly, it can increase the overall taste of a recipe.

Stevia is a plant-based, natural sweetener that has gained popularity over the past decade. It often shows up in flavored drinks, protein powders, and many other food products. Stevia will have zero effect on body-fat (0 calories) or blood sugar levels (0 glycemic index). If you have yet to use or consume stevia, start small for two reasons:
    1.   there have been reported allergic reactions (rarely of course, but again, use caution)

2. too much will ruin the taste of whatever you are adding it to (similar to artificial sweeteners)

Speaking of artificial sweeteners ... artificial sweeteners are also 0 calories and will not cause body-fat. They are also generally considered safe in regards to raising blood sugar. On the surface, they sound very similar to stevia.

However, studies claim that even though both stevia and artificial sweeteners are 0 calories (aka not digested and absorbed by the body), artificial sweeteners are in fact somewhat absorbed—as high as 15%. This raises red flags as many artificial sweeteners contain chlorine. Chlorine atoms are substituted into sucrose to create sucralose.

Whether you choose to ingest artificial sweeteners is up to you (check your chewing gum). Again, they will not cause body-fat or blood sugar issues, but there may be potential long term health issues. Whether you buy into the latter is your call.

As I mentioned before, honey is not Vegan. This is for a number of reasons. The first is the exploitation of bees. Bees put in a *massive* amount of work to produce honey, only for humans to steal it and replace it with an unhealthy alternative (for the bee). Bees are extremely important to the environment and the food chain! The extinction of bees would lead to the extinction of **countless** plants and animals. We are already killing them at an alarming rate!

Honey also contains digestive enzymes from the bee itself, as honey is produced through a consumption, and eventual regurgitation by the bee. Yes, honey is technically bee throw-up!

Again, every single form of processed sugar will lead to body-fat. Cut it out and your taste pallets will change. Fruit will taste far sweeter. Even natural peanut butter (*just* peanut butter) will begin to feel like a treat. And this isn't a bad thing. If natural peanut butter is considered a treat, your diet probably looks *pretty good* to say the least. And yes, every time I mention nut butters, I am assuming no sweeteners, hydrogenated oils, and the like. The ingredients should say something like "roasted almonds", or "roasted peanuts, salt", etc.

Yeast

An overgrowth of yeast in the body is known as "candida". Candida can cause a variety of conditions and symptoms: fatigue, brain fog, yeast infections, irritable bowel syndrome, acne, rashes, oral thrush, eczema, among others. Back in my meat-eating days, I experimented with a "candida elimination diet". I stayed on this diet for about two months. The diet called for:

- no sugar (sugar causes candida to multiply)
- no dairy
- no yeast (duh)
- no fermented foods
- initially no fruit, eventually "re-introducing" fruit

I was basically living on: meat, eggs, vegetables, as well as making pancakes with a clean (yeast-free, sugar-free, gluten-free) flour. Not the most exciting of diets by any means. Just weeks into the diet, my skin *completely* cleared up, my bowel movements normalized, and I just felt (overall) so much healthier. There obviously was something to this.

This diet changed the way I looked at food forever. While I did revert back to occasionally consuming yeast, sugar, and dairy, I started to pay extremely close attention to ingredient labels, and everything I was putting into my body. Overall, my diet became far healthier than prior to the cleanse.

Now obviously yeast was not the only ingredient I eliminated. Eliminating dairy and sugar **exponentially** improves overall health. However, even during times when I was not consuming dairy and sugar, and I did consume food items that contained yeast (bread, for example—even gluten-free bread), my acne returned, as did my stomach issues. This holds true for today, even while eating 100% Vegan.

I always hear people say, "stop eating bread and pasta" to lose body-fat. I can say that this statement is only half true. I have experimented time and time again with both food items.

The primary difference between the two food items is yeast. I eat brown rice (and other gluten-free) pasta every so often. I never have an issue with it. And why would I? All brown rice pasta is, is brown rice that was turned into flour, that was then turned into pasta. It is slightly more processed, however the ingredients and glycemic loads are identical.

This topic of yeast is also where my fear of fermented foods comes from. This is why I say to experiment with tempeh. Fermentation and yeast go hand-in-hand. I encourage you to pay very close attention to how certain ingredients and types of foods make you feel (and look).

Quick Story: When I was around 8 or 9 years old, my mother took me to a local doctor who claimed he could eliminate seasonal allergies. There was an article about him in the paper about all of the people he had been helping. I went to this guy two or three times. The appointment consisted of three parts. I forget the order, but one part was typical chiropractic adjustments of the neck and back. Another was this hand-held machine he used to "click and roll" up and down my spine.

The third portion of the appointment is why I am telling this story in the first place. The doctor would hand me a vial that contained a substance inside. He had all these different enclosed vials, each with a label. He would instruct me to clench my hand shut with the vial inside, while simultaneously raising the same side fist (and arm) upward against the downward pressure of his hand (as it gripped the top of my wrist). A strength test of sorts.

Long story short, the vial that produced the weakest strength response from myself was none other than the yeast vial. Each time. He sent me home with a yeast elimination diet that I completely disregarded. I thought he was a quack! Wouldn't you?

After my successful yeast elimination diet (over ten years later), I couldn't help but think back to this doctor and his wacky methods. I came to two potential conclusions:

Either:

1. His methods were legit. He found out I had an issue with yeast through his "strength tests".

Or

2. All along he knew that most humans consumed a high amount of sugar and yeast. And that giving a patient an elimination diet would improve his or her seasonal allergies. This would obviously mean that his methods (and all of the other vials) were a complete mirage. Then again, I guess it doesn't matter—results are results.

Gluten

Gluten refers to the proteins found in wheat, rye, barley, certain oats, and variations (and hybrids) of these food types (spelt, kamut, among others). "Gluten-free diets" became mainstream not long after the turn of the century. Everyone from professional athletes to average Joe's (and Jane's) boasted the benefits of this odd sounding diet. On a personal level, I have experimented with gluten-free diets quite a bit. From this, and researching independent cases, I have drawn a number of conclusions:

1. Some individuals are far more sensitive to gluten than others. To the point where it is a legit allergy. When these individuals went gluten-free, their lives changed for the better *dramatically*. It wasn't just "oh I feel like I have more energy". The difference was night and day.

2. For the majority of individuals, a little bit of gluten "here and there" is relatively harmless. I have seen people that claim to be gluten intolerant, unknowingly (and continually) eat products that contain gluten, and show zero signs of a potential allergy.

3. The amount consumed matters. It seems there is a threshold one can consume before symptoms occur. I came to this conclusion through my own experimentation. When I ate gluten sparingly, I did not notice a difference. When I purposely changed my primary carbohydrate sources to wheat-based, I began to experience bloating and digestive issues.

The easiest test to measure potential gluten intolerance is eating "seitan". In my opinion, seitan is the best tasting, and closest resembling "mock meat" out there. I have gone on seitan binges. It, however, is literally *pure gluten*. Eating a ton of seitan is not the same as eating a ton of wheat. It is essentially isolating the gluten from the meat, and then consuming it in a far higher quantity and concentration.

When I eat seitan, I break out in acne and my stomach "goes bonkers" consistently. I wish this were not the case, as again: when dressed up properly, seitan is delicious. It is also lean and high in protein (it is protein after all). Eating wheat here and there does not do much to set me off. Pushing this into overdrive by consuming high amounts of pure gluten and BAM—three zits on my face within a day or two (with otherwise clean eating).

Do not take my word for it. I encourage you to perform the same experiments as me. With not only gluten, but yeast as well. One thing I will mention is this: I am of the opinion that yeast is worse for humans than gluten (outside of a legit gluten allergy). Yet we always hear about gluten-free diets, but we rarely hear of yeast-free diets.

Drugs

Drugs will have a massive impact on any diet. I am not just referring to "hard drugs". Even socially acceptable drugs such as: caffeine, alcohol, and antibiotics can wreak havoc on a diet. I will simply list a few variations of drugs and the effects they can have on aspects of a diet. Keep in mind that I am not covering all types of drugs. My goal is to get you to pay attention to how certain drugs affect factors such as appetite and digestion.

Caffeine
Caffeine is extremely good at suppressing hunger. An individual could go five, six, hours of zero appetite after consuming caffeine. As you will learn in the next chapter, this is not a good problem to have. Even if your goal is lowering body-fat, you should be eating (on average) every three hours. This is especially true if you engage regularly in resistance exercise.

If you do choose to consume caffeine, I recommend trying it one of these three ways:

1. Consume it immediately before eating. This way the caffeine will not kick in until you are pretty much already finished with your meal. You got it in on your preferred empty stomach, your meal is finished, and you now have ~three hours until your next meal.

2. Consume it during, or right after eating. Same concept at number 1, minus the empty stomach. Next meal in ~three hours.

3. Force yourself (as a habit/ritual) to consume the meal about an hour after the caffeine. This way, the caffeine has two hours to wean off before your next meal, and the prior meal will have more time to move through digestion. The coffee will kick in quicker and stronger than if eaten on a full stomach.

Caffeine can also speed things up a bit too much in terms of digestion. It is very common for too much caffeine to result in some form of mild diarrhea. This should obviously be kept in mind— especially when leaving the house or consuming at work (or better yet, before a workout).

Medical Marijuana

You obviously already know where I am going with this one. Yes, marijuana (THC) is a *massive* appetite stimulant. To the point where an individual can have a huge meal, inhale the plant, and minutes later crave a meal (often, sweets). It doesn't take a genius to figure out how this can cause someone to have an issue adhering to a diet. But don't worry—there are tricks to work around the appetite stimulation.

1. Do not use marijuana right before eating. This can cause you to overeat or crave something that you should not be eating. The only exception would be to stimulate hunger because something else **legitimately** depressed it (e.g. cancer patients and nausea—people who truly need it).

2. Do not use marijuana right after eating. This can cause you to feel very sluggish. This can cause complacency and "laying around". It should not be used to relax. Relaxing should always be a natural process. Using a drug to get there can cause the body to require it. Requiring a drug to relax = anxiety.

   Using marijuana right after eating can also cause you to feel hungry again. This can obviously lead to another meal (a massive amount of calories in a short amount of time ... aka body-fat).

Use it roughly an hour after eating. Therefore, your food will be further along through digestion and you will still have 2 hours to use your medication (productively) before you have to eat again. Also, do not have sweets around. This is not just a "weed thing". Don't buy them, period. If they aren't there, you can't eat them.

Marijuana can also cause constipation. This is especially true if used shortly after waking up (before your first bowel movement). This can cause you to be "backed up", which will lead to fatigue and nausea, among other symptoms throughout the day.

Opiates and Opioids
Opiates and opioids refer to narcotic pain-killers that act on opiate receptors in the brain. Codeine, oxycodone, hyrdrocodone, morphine, tramadol, among others. These types of drugs suppress hunger even worse than caffeine. I won't go into too much detail on this one. Just know that you are probably going to have to force yourself to eat at some point. **These drugs are not meant to be used long-term.** Also, do not use another drug (such as marijuana) to "get back" the hunger. This is a slippery slope.

Opiates and opoids are also notorious for constipation. If you find yourself in a situation where you have to take them (post-surgery, etc), try not to dose until after your first bowel movement. If your first "BM" is taking too long to occur, chug an extra glass or two of water.

Anti-inflammatories

Another quickie. Anti-inflammatories are known to cause an upset stomach. Pain, to gas, to potentially diarrhea. They can also contribute to a potential ulcer. Do not consume them on an empty stomach. I would suggest after consuming a moderately sized meal. Generally speaking, they will not have a major effect on appetite.

Antibiotics

Antibiotics can (and will) throw off your whole digestive system. This often leads to nausea, lack of hunger, and potentially diarrhea. There are suggestions out there to take a probiotic while taking an antibiotic to "replenish the 'good' bacteria the antibiotic kills off". I honestly cannot tell you the last time I took an antibiotic, but I can tell you that I am not a probiotic person. I have had issues with them in the past. I like to let my body adjust itself through clean, nutritious eating and drinking tons of water. What you choose to do here is completely up to you. The suggestion is to take the probiotic a few hours after the antibiotic.

Alcohol

I think it goes without saying that alcohol is a non-compliant ingredient. Alcohol is literally poison to the body. I won't go into much detail here. Just try to limit alcohol to special occasions and do not go overboard.

3 When And How To Eat

Creating A Meal Schedule

Meal timing is essential to accomplishing dietary goals. Without a meal schedule, it is extremely easy to lose track of when you have last eaten, and when you should be eating again. From a general health point of view, this is not the biggest deal in the world. However, from a goal oriented point of view (strength gain, fat loss, muscle gain, aesthetics, weight loss, etc), this is a huge deal.

Let me preface by saying that I am not going to get into any science to back this. There is no need to go up this alley as this work has already been done by scores of successful individuals over the past "x" amount of years. We are simply going to model these individuals.

I will address "Eating For A Specific Goal" at the latter end of this chapter. For now, let's look at the ideology of a meal schedule itself.

As I stated above, a meal schedule is necessary to remind yourself when it is time to eat. No different than a work schedule or daily planner. In fact, the meal schedule should be tailored *into* your everyday schedule to ensure that it is practical to repeat on a daily basis. It needs to be written down, typed up, entered into your phone, or whatever method you prefer that keeps the information at your fingertips. Life is crazy and unpredictable … I promise you: **if you attempt to create this schedule mentally (and only mentally), you will falter and eventually fall off completely.**

Here is an example of a meal schedule, tied into a daily schedule for a nine-to-five office worker.

Gym Day (Mon/Wed/Fri)

7am: Wake up | Glass or bottle of water | Vitamin B-12
½ cup Oats w/ blueberries , Some spinach on side ,
1 scoop protein in water , Vitamin D-3
Cup of coffee with almond milk

7:30am: Brush, Shower, Get ready for work

8am: Make a double portion of protein smoothies in blender | Drink another water

8:20am: Leave for work

10:15am: *Drink smoothie #1* |
                        |---> Drink water throughout
1:30pm: *Drink smoothie #2* |

5:20pm: Tofu stir fry: 1 block tofu, 1 tbsp olive oil, broccoli, garlic powder, black pepper
1 cup brown rice pasta

5:40pm: *Eat ½ of Stir fry* | Drink another water

6:30pm: Go to the gym for 1hr | Drink another water

8:00pm: Shower

8:20pm: *Eat rest of stir fry* | Drink another water

10:00pm: Sleep

You will notice that this meal schedule addresses more than just "when to eat". Cooking time is also taken into consideration. Water intake as well, among other activities. Your meal schedule does not need to be this rigid or detailed. It just needs to work for you.

Every single meal in the schedule is self prepared. However, each meal is quick and simple. The oats can take anywhere from 5 to 10 minutes (depending on quick cooking oats vs. standard rolled oats). The smoothie is a double portion and takes 10 minutes tops (an average of 5 minutes per meal). A simple tofu stir fry takes about 20 minutes, 25 minutes tops. Over two portions, this is just over ten minutes per meal. Five meals, ~40 minutes of cooking and preparation. This number can be even lower if the stir fry is substituted for something quicker.

This is ~forty minutes a day to:
1. achieve your goal / dream body / feel awesome about yourself
2. eat healthy, increase energy, avoid & reverse disease, live longer, feel awesome physically

The vast majority of "westerners" spend far more time:
1. watching TV
2. browsing the internet & social media
3. snacking on junk food
4. stressing
5. playing video games

There are also techniques discussed in the next chapter (Chapter 4) that can lower this 40 minute cook/prep time even more. For example: Batch/Bulk Cooking

Take a look at the meal schedule again and notice the timing of each meal.

Meal 1: ~7:15am
Meal 2: ~10:15am *+3 hours*
Meal 3: ~1:30pm *+3 hours and 15min*
Meal 4: ~5:40pm *+4 hours and 10min*
Meal 5: ~8:20pm *+2 hours and 40min*

On average, each meal is ~3 hours and 15 minutes apart. On this diet plan, we subscribe to the "3-hour rule".

The 3-hour rule is not an exact science. It is to serve as a guideline that can be adjusted based upon an individual's current goals, activity level, metabolism, and times when one just cannot eat (due to certain priorities). You can also think of it as the "3-hour rule, plus or minus 30 minutes". Again, I will touch on this more when I address "Eating For A Specific Goal" at the latter end of this chapter.

This rule is not just for bodybuilders! I hear this all the time … "I am not trying to look like a bodybuilder, so why should I eat like one?!" Everyone has this image of a tanned, oiled up, muscular man or woman on a stage flexing. Yes, these are types of bodybuilders. However:

1. prototypical bodybuilders also train a certain way in regards to resistance exercise/programming.. they prioritize muscle hypertrophy (muscle gaining), while minimizing body-fat over everything else … it is a sport/competition

2. they take dieting to a whole new level in order to look that lean and muscular … it doesn't happen by accident! … again, it is a sport/competition

3. the ones that are *insanely* massive (think "Mr. Universe") are unnatural (steroids, pro-hormones, etc)

Saying this, elite bodybuilders are masters of eating. Masters of the ability to gain and maintain lean muscle while shedding body-fat.

Even if you have zero intention of looking like a bodybuilder and your goal is simply to "look in better shape", the quickest and most efficient way to get there is by eating like a bodybuilder. *Even* as a 100lb female that wants to "tone up for the summer" – the quickest and most efficient way to accomplish this is by eating like a bodybuilder.

"Macro"-ing

macro-nutrient: Fats, Carbohydrates, and Protein

Now that you have an idea of what a meal schedule can look like, let's tackle exactly *how* to create each individual meal. In this section, I will also address "Eating For A Specific Goal" and modifying the 3-hour rule.

Remember the Food List from Chapter 1? How it was broken down into 5 categories (fats, carbs, proteins, fruits, and veggies)? We will now go over how to build meals from the foods on the list. This is going to be an extremely easy concept to grasp.

As I stated in Chapter 1, several food items can dip into multiple categories. I gave the example of beans containing a relatively high amount of protein, but not necessarily being a lean source of protein (meaning that eating too many could lead to an increase in body fat). Again, beans contain a significant amount of calories from complex carbohydrates as well. This same notion applies to nuts and fat content.

Saying this, we are going to look at two ways of building meals:

1. Building meals heading with a "lean" source of protein
2. Building meals heading with a "not as lean" source of protein

First, let's take a look at some common sources of Plant Protein:

Per 100 Calories			
Food Item	Carbohydrates(g)	Fat(g)	Protein(g)
Avg. Protein Powder	~2	~2	20
Spinach	15	2	13
Tofu	2.5	6	10

Food Item	Carbohydrates(g)	Fat(g)	Protein(g)
Tempeh*	6	6	10
Broccoli	20	2	8
Soybeans	6	6	10
Lentils	18	0	9
Kidney Bean	18	0	7
Kale	20	2	6
Chickpeas (Garbanzo Beans)	17	1.5	5.5

*Again, tempeh is fermented–I do not eat it. Feel free to experiment. Also not on the list: seitan aka vital wheat gluten (very high in protein, however it is pure gluten)

Let me explain this table very quickly. Immediately, I must mention that 100 calories of kale, spinach, and broccoli is a *very* large amount of greens. So while each contains a decent amount of protein *per calorie*, it isn't exactly realistic to consume that much in one sitting. I am sure that there are individuals out there that do this, but it does not really go along with the theme of this book.

Moreover, do not get too caught up in comparing the numbers in each column to each other. Not all proteins are the same (amino-acid content, complete vs incomplete, etc). Not all carbohydrates are the same (simple vs complex vs coming from leafy greens, etc). And not all fats are the same (Monounsaturated vs. Polyunsaturated vs. Saturated). More on this is a bit.

1. <u>Building meals heading with a "lean" source of protein:</u>

When a lean source of protein is at the head, it is necessary to add either a fat or carbohydrate source to the meal. The reason is very simple: if you just eat lean protein, it will immediately burn up, the meal will fail to provide lasting energy, and your hunger will return very quickly. (The meal will also not be very nutritious.)

Think of meal-building as this:

Protein + a carb or fat + a green (or lesser veggie) = a complete meal

On this diet plan, the lean proteins I have listed are Tofu, Tempeh, and Plant Protein Powder. Again, these are not the only lean sources of plant protein. Seitan (vital wheat gluten) is also lean from a nutrition label perspective. However, its healthiness is disputable. If you absolutely love seitan, and your body has handled it well, have at it. Just as I said to experiment with tempeh. **Remember, you do not have to eat like me**—I am simply giving you a <u>guideline</u>. Spirulina and chlorella are also very high in protein. They also smell and taste like fish food. Again, not for me. If you like them and your body handles them well, go for it.

I prefer Tofu and Protein Powder. Tofu is made from soybeans. The beans are processed in a way that separates the "soy milk" portion from the fiber and hull. The milk portion is then mixed with a coagulating agent (such as calcium sulfate, magnesium chloride, and/or nigari) and eventually processed into the blocks we all identify with tofu. Why do I love it?

1. It's decently lean and high in protein.
2. It's delicious, versatile, and mentally it replaces meat (I ate meat until age 23).
3. It's widely available at stores and Asian restaurants.

The only negative is that it's amino-acid profile is not exactly the richest. While the processing of the soybean into tofu "leans it out", it also results in a loss of some amino-acids. However, food combining dampens any worry of coming up deficient in any amino-acids.

And then there is Protein Powder ... there are many individuals out there that will bash the idea of considering a supplement as an integral part of a nutrition plan. However, the fact is this: Protein Powder is undoubtedly the leanest and richest (from an amino-acid perspective) protein source a Vegan can possibly eat. I have experimented with protein powders for over a decade. The majority are clean and have zero effect on fat gain, stomach issues, acne, and all of the other problems that come with maximally processed foods.

Moreover, you can put protein powder in pretty much anything, including a small glass of water. Nothing is quicker or more versatile. It is an absolute godsend at increasing the taste of green smoothies. It is illogical to not have protein powder in your pantry at all times. Even meat-eaters use it!

The fact is this, outside of leafy greens (and spirulina/chlorella), there is no such thing as a legitimately, high nutrition source of protein. It does not exist. So to bash protein powder because of its "lack of nutrition" is just flat out silly. One should view protein as **fulfilling a macro-nutrient requirement.** Paramount nutrition comes from GREENS, and to a lesser extent, other vegetables and fruits.

Which brings us to the next step in meal-building: Leafy Greens. Each meal, you should strive to include leafy greens (spinach, kale, broccoli, etc). These are the most nutrient dense foods on the face of the earth. I prefer spinach, kale, and broccoli (all high in vitamins A, C, K, calcium, and protein, among others). If leafy greens are not available during a certain meal, try for a "lesser" vegetable such as carrots (high in vitamin A) or cauliflower (high in vitamin c) – these are just two examples. If vegetables are not available, look to fruits such as berries and the like.

How much can you eat? If it is a leafy green, unlimited. In fact, **the more, the better**. The same goes for anything in the vegetable column on the Food List. You can get away with a hefty amount of fruit as well, but I wouldn't go overboard—especially as it gets closer to bedtime.

So far, you have a lean protein source and a high nutrition source (preferably leafy greens). These two combined would be enough for a quick meal or snack before bed. However, to create a satiating meal that provides a legitimate energy source for a few hours, you need to add a food item from the Fat column or Carbohydrate column on the Food List.

If you choose a Fat, shoot for one serving. Keep in mind: the number of calories in one serving of fat are not the same for each fat source. For example:

-1 serving of extra virgin coconut oil (1 tbsp) is ~130 calories*, 14g of fat (12 of which is saturated fat)
-1 serving of natural peanut butter (2 tbsp) is ~190 calories*, 16g of fat (8 of which is monounsaturated, 5 polyunsaturated)

*note, some coconut oils are 120 calories, some nut butters go up to 210 calories per serving

Do not worry about the calories or grams of fat—just measure out one serving. As you can see, fats are extremely caloric. Play it safe and use a TBSP measure to ensure you do not go overboard (assuming you are using a nut butter or oil). If you are using nuts themselves, read the nutrition label and find out what a serving is. Most nuts are ¼ cup per serving, but be sure to double check.

If you choose a carbohydrate, measure it by the calories. Depending on your goal, this number can be anywhere from 100-200+ calories per serving. For example:

-1/2 cup of rolled oats is usually around 170-190 calories
-1/4 cup of brown rice (dry, before cooking) is 150 calories

As you can see there is a bit of measuring/portioning involved in this diet. This really only affects the initial stages of the diet and it will never become as intense as (say) weighing your food.

By this point, you have your lean protein source, your nutrition source (leafy greens!), and either your carb or fat source. The only facet I have not mentioned is the one-million dollar Vegan question: *How much protein!?* Honestly, this is very goal dependent, but if I had to give a universal answer, shoot for ~20g+ per meal. And this 20g does not *all* need to come from the protein source. I am talking 20+ grams from the protein, the greens, and either the carb or fat source. Your lean protein source should be at least 100 calories, more than likely 120-200. Just know this, a lean protein will never be the cause of body-fat gain. However, overeating food items from the carbohydrate or fat columns on the Food List will cause an increase in body-fat.

Looking at the meal as a whole:
- Your protein sources can range from ~100-200 calories (~150 on average).
- Your fat sources (one serving) can range from ~120-210 calories (~165 calories on average).
- Depending on your goal, your carbohydrate sources can range from 100-200+ calories (150 on average).
- And not that anyone counts vegetable calories, but I would estimate anywhere from 25-50 calories (~37.5 on average).

What number should we be shooting for per meal? Again, this is goal dependent, just like the 3-hour rule. Generally speaking, somewhere between 350-400 calories per meal. In the third section of this chapter, I will finally address how to determine "where you should be at" depending on your goal, as well as when you should choose a carbohydrate versus a fat (in terms of meal building).

This is the way I eat, and really is the basis of this book (time-saving, minimal effort). The majority of my meals take only 5-10 minutes of preparation. I simply view each meal as:

1. not consuming culprit foods and ingredients
2. fulfilling macro-nutrient requirements in acceptable proportions (numbers)
3. and adding a leafy green

Here are a few of my staple meals from using this model:

Protein Smoothie ~5-7 minutes
-1 scoop protein powder mixed in water and/or almond/cashew milk (~120-150 cal 21g protein)
-2 tbsp natural peanut butter (~190 cal 16g fat 8g protein 7g carb)
-frozen strawberries + either mixed berries or mixed tropical fruit (1-2 servings depending on space in smoothie cup)
-as much kale or spinach as I can fit
~375 cal ~31g protein 1 serving of fat , however many carbs is in the fruit and leafy greens (I do not count carbs from fruit and veggies)

Tofu Stir Fry (makes 2 servings) ~20 minutes, 10minute/serving
-1 block tofu (400 cal 40g protein) ... seasoned with garlic powder, black pepper, etc
-1 tbsp extra virgin olive oil for pan 120cal 14g fat
-brown rice pasta or other gluten-free pasta ~200cal 41g carb 4g protein
-generous amount of broccoli
-if time, ½ a white onion
per serving: ~380 cal 25g protein ½ serving fat 100cal worth of pasta

Dry Roasted Edamame or Peanut Butter w/ Protein Powder & Raw Spinach/Broccoli/or Kale <5 minutes
-1 scoop protein powder (~120 cal 21g protein)
-2 tbsp natural peanut butter (~190 cal 16g fat 8g protein 7g carb) OR 150-200 cal (~1/3 to 1/2 cup) worth of dry roasted edamame (13g to 18g protein, 4g to 7g fat, 11g to 17g carb)
-Raw Spinach/Broccoli/or Kale ... If spinach or kale, crumple leaves, try not to taste, chew until broken down, wash down with water.
*per serving: ~300-350 cal | **31g to 41g protein** | either 1 serving of fat or 100-200 cal worth of carbs*

*Can substitute edamame with gluten-free oats/pasta, roasted chickpeas, canned beans, etc... peanut butter with any other serving of fat (almonds, coconut oil (1 tbsp), etc)

2. <u>Building meals heading with a "not as lean" source of protein:</u>

Next, we will look at building meals with a "not as lean" source of protein at the head. On this diet plan, I recommend that this source be some type of bean: kidney beans, black beans, mung beans, garbanzo beans (chickpeas), cannelloni beans, lentils, soybeans, and the like. As we have discussed, beans contain a generous amount of protein. They are also very versatile and can be put in: soups and stews, salads, stir-fries, wraps—they can even be made into dips (black bean dip, hummus, etc).

Let's jump right into "macro-ing" these types of meals.

Your protein source is also going to be your carbohydrate source, or at least a large portion of it. The overall meal is still going to be ~350-400calories, with the goal of ~20+ grams of protein. Keep in mind that these meals can exceed 400 calories. This is especially true if a large portion of the meal is greens & veggies. I am just giving you a bench mark to start at, as I am for pretty much every number found in this book.

Naturally, these meals will contain less fat. Adding significant fat calories to an already carb-heavy meal can result in a body-fat gain.

I still prefer to limit these meals to ~200 calories worth of food items from the carbohydrate column (in this case, the beans). However, I also do not dip much under 200 calories either, as I want to keep the protein content as high as possible. You can also split these 200 calories between beans and another food item from the carbohydrate column such as rice or sweet potatoes.

Beans and rice have complimentary amino-acid profiles and are a very popular combination. However, as far as this diet is concerned, try to ensure that the majority of this combination still comes from the beans portion. Beans are much higher in protein than rice. Not to sound "protein-crazy", but there are certain lifestyles that *do* call for higher protein intake. Not to mention the transitioning meat eaters that are accustomed to higher protein diets. Even if it is unnecessary, it provides peace of mind that these individuals are getting enough protein on a Vegan diet.

At this point, you have your protein and carbohydrate columns taken care of and are ~200 calories into the meal-build. What about fats? You really don't need to add much fat to these meals, if at all. Like I said, too many calories from carbohydrates and fats (in one sitting) can lead to a gain in body-fat. If you do choose to add a fat to this type of meal, keep it to ~1/3 a serving to ½ tops. Feel free to experiment and keep an eye on how this affects your body composition over time. Avocados and extra virgin olive oil are two sources of fat that often accompany beans, rice, and/or sweet potatoes in a dish.

Rounding out these meals will be an assortment of vegetables. As always, prioritize the leafy greens: spinach, kale, and broccoli. However, you also have more breathing room (regarding calories) to add even more items from the vegetable column. Onions, peppers, carrots, cauliflower—whichever vegetables you prefer. If you haven't noticed by now, this is a more traditional way of Vegan eating. (We are just keeping track of macro-nutrient counts.) These meals contain tons of color, veggies of all sorts, and only "whole foods".

It is still very easy to hit that ~20g of protein mark with this type of eating. 200 calories worth of soybeans alone is 20g. Same with mung beans. 200 calories of lentils is 18g. Kidney beans 14g, black beans 13g, chickpeas 11g. However, 200 calories worth of brown rice is just 5g of protein. So keep this in mind when substituting a portion of beans for rice. (200 calories-worth of sweet potatoes is ~4g of protein.)

This type of eating is less clear-cut than the former in regards to gaining muscle and losing body-fat. It may take a bit more experimentation to find meal combinations that line up with your goals. Start with my recommendation of 200 calories worth of beans, add in your leafy greens and enough food items from the vegetable column to fill you up. Remember, all of this is clean eating. As long as you avoid culprit foods and ingredients from chapter 2, you are three-quarters there. The rest is self-control and second grade math.

The reason I am showing specific protein and calorie counts is many individuals have goals beyond just "eating healthy and not being overweight". In order for Veganism to spread to the masses, there needs to be more Vegan: professional athletes, strongmen and women, gymnasts, dancers, bodybuilders, models, power-lifters and the like. The fact is, a large portion of society does not believe it is possible to achieve the same results on a Vegan diet than on a non-Vegan diet. Even though there are current examples of Vegans in all of these categories, there are not enough.

This is one of my chief aims of this book. There are way too many Vegan books out there that are just recipe money-grabs. They do not address topics such as meal timing and macro-ing—vital information for any diet! It is no wonder that so many Vegans feel lost, eat unhealthy, gain weight, and potentially revert back to a meat-eating diet.

Eating For A Specific Goal

As I have stated several times in this chapter, the numbers that appear in this book will be need to be adjusted depending on your goal(s). "I want to lose weight." "I want to get jacked." "I want to get lean and ripped." "I want to look like a swimsuit model." "I have to get to 300lbs to play on the offensive line." – I want to address *everything*.

1. Prioritizing A Low Body-Fat % While Gaining Lean Muscle
This is by far the most common case, so I will spend the most time on it. Obviously, the amount of muscle individuals want to gain can vary (e.g. a bodybuilder vs. a swimsuit model), but *pretty much* everyone wants to be relatively lean and have some amount of lean muscle. I don't think it is a stretch to make this statement!

First off, these individuals must partake in some sort of resistance training. Be it: weights, gymnastics, simple calisthenics—something! Muscle needs a reason to grow in the first place.

Resistance training also increases metabolism, burns calories, optimizes hormone levels, and gives one "more breathing room" as far as how much he or she can cheat and remain lean.

Overall, the diet also has to be on-point. The stricter one adheres to the guidelines, the quicker he or she will gain muscle, lose body-fat, and accomplish his or her goal. It is a very straightforward concept. The guidelines are everything we have gone over so far:

- eating the right foods (Chapter 1), not eating culprit foods (Chapter 2)
- timing meals properly (this chapter)
- proportioning/macro-ing meals correctly (this chapter)

A lean physique requires consistent clean eating. Now obviously "lean" is a relative term. For some individuals, lean simply means "not overweight". The other extreme is professional bodybuilders (the ones that get on stage and pose). The elite of this group eat pretty much 100% compliant. 90% compliance to bodybuilders does not mean 9 out of 10 perfect meals. 90% means 9 perfect meals, the 10th meal is perfect, outside of that inch of tofu that was eaten ten minutes early. Of course I am exaggerating here, but my point is, these individuals have *extremely* high standards when it comes to eating. Again, they do not look like this by accident. I am talking extremes to give a clear picture of what it takes to achieve a certain result.

90% compliance to other individuals may mean 9 perfect meals, 1 cheat meal. This group of people will still be on their way to a lean physique and good health. This, assuming the cheat meal is not 4000 calories worth of sugar and culprit foods/ingredients. (I will touch more on cheat meals in Chapter 5).

70% compliance should honestly be the bare minimum. Less than this means the individual associates food more with pleasure (a drug) than fuel (health/results). Seek pleasure elsewhere! And again, standards are everything. 70% does not necessarily mean 7 out of 10 perfect meals. 70% could simply mean:

"I had an average day eating … I ate 6 meals—5 were perfect, however I ate two of them too close together, and the second meal also contained a piece of bread".

Five out of six is 83%. However, the meal timing was off and bread (assuming it is not yeast free/gluten free) is a non-compliant food on this diet (hence the "70%"). Let me make this clear: **a bad enough cheat can kill even 2 days of perfect eating.** This is something that needs to be remembered consistently!

Now, how should these individuals time their meals? This can depend on a number of factors. 3 hours is the beginning guideline. When is it okay to lower this number?

1. You are working out a ton and getting extremely hungry even after waiting just 2 and a half hours. Eat! Your muscles need to be fed. If not, the body will fail to fuel them and they will fail to grow/disappear. Keep in mind that hungry means "I need food" – not "man, I could go for a protein shake right now, they are so good!" If you are unsure about whether you are actually hungry or simply craving something, ask yourself, "Would I eat broccoli right now?" Seriously. And if you still aren't sure, make the meal and **eat the greens first**, then the protein, then the carb or fat.

2. Your prior meal was too small. For whatever reason: you were in a rush, lack of food on hand, etc. Obviously this will cause hunger to arise quicker!

3. Your muscles are very sore from workouts. I am talking legit muscle soreness. Not fatigue, not joint pain. "DOMS" as they call it: **d**elayed **o**nset **m**uscle **s**oreness. You deadlifted on Tuesday and your hamstrings and butt have been sore from Wednesday to Friday. This will absolutely increase hunger! Same concept as number 1.

When should the 3-hour rule exceed 3 hours? Pretty much the opposite: You don't work out (or do very little). Your metabolism is slow. Your hormones are off. Your last meal was too large and you still are not hungry. You get where I am going with this. It may be best to space meals by 3 and a half to 4 hours.

Also, (as mentioned in Chapter 2) keep in mind that certain drugs can put off the hunger feeling. Caffeine and opiates/opioids (pain-killers) are notorious for this. If you are an individual that must have caffeine at certain points of the day, time it so that it does not interfere with hunger levels. Perhaps drink the coffee immediately after eating. Or try 30-60 minutes after if you prefer an emptier stomach. Try not to exceed that an hour. Caffeine can easily curb hunger for 3-4+ hours! Opiates and opioids are even worse! Please take all of this into consideration.

How about macro-ing and portion sizes? The reasons are pretty much the same as the meal timing reasons. If you work out quite a bit, your meals can be a bit larger. This does not mean eating 400 calories worth of carbs or fat in one sitting instead of ~150-200. However, it may mean 50 to 100 calories extra. Or perhaps 10-20 more grams of protein (if you think you need it). Or better yet, even more vegetables—*especially* if the main goal is leaning out (getting cut/toned).

This will obviously take some experimenting! The guidelines are there to minimize this. Keep in mind that eating a certain way for one day, will not show the next day. It will take at least an extra day or two to see a visible result (depending on a number of factors). I recommend testing portion and timing sizes over at least 1 week, preferably 2. **The "checker" is looking in the mirror or taking progress pictures!** *Do not go by the scale!*

The number on the scale is just a number. Dehydration techniques (alone) can cause a 20lb+ "loss" in just days—grapplers and fighters purposely do this before matches to "make weight", only to re-hydrate the weight the very next day. STOP living by that number! Look in the mirror! Better yet, take a picture of yourself each day for a week or two. Has your physique improved? It has? Great! Keep it up. It hasn't? Or not at the rate you expect? Fiddle with the numbers! Individuals that are trying to gain or maintain a lean, muscular, toned physique should be eating at least 4 meals a day, preferably 5 or 6. By the way, "lean" does not equate to skinny or frail … lean refers to low body-fat % … you can be lean and 200lbs+!

Six meals may sound like overkill, but remember, we are only looking at ~350-450 calories per meal. Less meals does not result in lower body-fat. More often it is the opposite. This is especially true if you work out. We want to fuel our muscles consistently. All while **only consuming clean foods, and consuming them in an amount that *does not* exceed the ideal amount that we need to achieve our goal.** This is how to build muscle and shed body-fat at the same time.

Try to eat within an hour of waking up. If you plan a morning fast once in a while to "give things a rest", go for it. However, this does not equate to improving your physique. During that fast, your muscles are starved. Do this too often, and you will lose/fail to gain muscle—essentially wasting workouts and periods of prior compliant eating that gained the muscle in the first place.

Do not be afraid to eat right before bedtime. As long as you are following all the rules of the diet, go for it. Just try not to make this meal high in fruit or food items from the carbohydrate list. Pick a protein, veggies, and a serving of fat. This meal can also be just protein and veggies.

As far as the decision to choose a food item from the Carbohydrate column versus a food item from the Fat column ... this is also goal and activity level-dependent. Generally speaking, place carbs closer to high-level physical activity: the meal before, or perhaps both meals before. Or one of the two meals before just to "get them in your system". The meal after is a potential choice as well. This is not something that really needs to be obsessed over for the average person. Even if you just decided to alternate meals: Carb Column, Fat Column, Carb Column, Fat Column, etc—this would work just fine.

And this isn't to say that even going an entire day of Carb Column (each meal) would be a reason to gain fat. Carb versus Fat is secondary to clean eating, timing, macro-ing, and portioning. Though I will say that a day of "all Fat Column" (no carbs) may cause you to be hungrier throughout the day.

Bodybuilders do use a technique termed "carb cycling" where they have specific amounts of carbs that they eat on certain days. High carb days, low carb days, 0 carb days, etc. Again, this is referring to food items from the Carbohdrate column (beans, rice, oats, sweet potatoes, etc). There are a number of variations of carb cycling out there. Some do high carb on weight lifting days, low carb on cardio or off days. Some start low carb day 1, and work up to a higher number by day ~5 (for example). Again, it is goal and program dependent. And honestly, unless your goal is to get "stage-level shredded", it isn't necessary. It isn't even necessary for that. Eat clean, time it right, macro it right, don't overeat.

2. Prioritizing Strength, Muscle Mass, & Weight Over Body-Fat
This individual still eats the same types of food. However, missing a meal, or being late to a meal is not an option. There is no "going hungry" on this plan. The 3-hour rule is pretty much the ceiling in regards to how long to wait in between meals. Meals themselves will often exceed that 1 serving of fat, or 200 calories-worth of carbohydrates. Protein may go up as well.

Fasting is not an option. Wake up → eat. Also, eat as close to bed as possible. Shoot, if you really want to go nuts: put some food next to your bed → go to sleep → set an alarm midway through the night → wake up → eat the food → go back to sleep. This is *complete* overkill for 99% of the population. However, some individuals who are really committed to putting on mass actually do this.

There is of course less concern in terms of cheat meals. However, eating "dirty" foods is completely unnecessary. Eat more food, more often, and do not go hungry. The amount of food intake versus the individual's activity level will determine how much muscle and fat is put on in the process.

3. Attaining A Low Body-Fat % Without Working Out
This individual needs to do **everything** in number 1, but to an even higher level of perfection. Not working out equates to a slow(er) metabolism, low level of muscle tone, sub-optimal hormone levels, and an inability to burn a high number of calories.

Here is a short summary of the chapter for quick reference:

- Write your meal schedule down. Incorporate it into life/work schedule and keep in mind prep time/cook time.
- Drink tons of water throughout the day.
- The 3-hour rule: Eat every 3 hours +/- 30min (or so) depending on goals, and activity level.
- If heading a meal with tofu, protein powder, or tempeh (or seitan, if you so choose):
  - Each meal = protein column + carbohydrate OR fat column (or a split) + veggies (greens!)
  - Shoot for 20+ grams of protein from 100-200 calories. 1 serving of fat or 100-200+ calories from complex carbohydrates (beans, rice, sweet potatoes, oats, etc). Greens (spinach, kale, broccoli, etc) or other veggies if greens are not available. The next option is fruit.
- If heading a meal with a bean (as the protein source):
  - Each Meal = ~200+ calories from beans + very little fat (if any) + greens and veggies
  - A portion of the beans' calories can be substituted for a grain (rice, etc) or sweet potatoes/yams. Again, more traditional vegan eating.
- Eat 4-6 meals per day. 350-450 calories (potentially more) per meal, depending on goals, activity level.
- The more you work out, the more you can eat, the more you can cheat and stay lean.
- If bulking, meals will (generally) be closer together and calories will increase.
- If looking to lean out (and gain, maintain muscle), try to eat as perfect as possible. The foods, the timing, the portions, the macro-ing.
- Test diet numbers in 1 week, to 2 week increments. Anything less is too small of a sample size.
- Do not use your scale to judge progress. Use a mirror or camera. Results will not appear over night.

4 Meal Preparation

This chapter is going to be extremely short. I just had to fit it in somewhere!

Meal preparation refers to anything that speeds up the process of cooking or consuming meals. Before we get into techniques such as "batch cooking", let's address a few concepts that are of equal importance.

Staples And Simplicity

Every successful dieter has a variety of "go-to" meals (staples). This is important for a number of reasons:

1. A go-to meal is obviously a meal that is enjoyable by the dieter. Taste is extremely important when it comes to long-term adherence to a diet.
2. Cooking or preparing said meals becomes quicker and easier, as the individual is constantly "practicing" the same steps during its creation (and coming up with more efficient processes).
3. Shopping also becomes simpler, as the individual knows exactly what he or she needs to purchase from the store. This also opens up the door for buying in bulk.

If this diet is far off from your current diet, it will take a bit of experimenting before you come up with a few staples. Think of what types of foods you enjoy (check the food list). What types of spices. What type of equipment you have (stove, oven, blender, etc). Keep in mind that this experimental period may be a bit rough. Recipes will be botched. Ingredients may even go to waste. This is OK. You will figure it out over time.

The best piece of advice I can give you is to come up with multiple meals that share a majority of the same ingredients. This will make shopping, storage, and preparation far simpler. Moreover, come up with meals that do not use too many ingredients. Avoid recipes that call for a "laundry-list" of food items. Save these for special occasions. Keep the rest simple!

My pantry, fridge, and freezer always look the same:

Freezer: frozen fruit, frozen kale or spinach, pre-made wraps (gluten-free flour, water, ev olive oil)
Fridge: cashew/almond milk, fresh kale, spinach, and/or broccoli, tofu
Pantry/counter: peanut butter, protein powder, gluten-free flour, extra virgin olive oil, extra virgin coconut oil, dry roasted edamame, gluten-free pasta, oats, garlic powder, basil, black pepper
Occasionally: Thai coconut milk, curry paste, agave or coconut sugar, nuts, fresh fruit, onions, coffee, crushed tomatoes, rice cakes

That's it—my diet is extremely simple, straight-forward, and everything tastes awesome to me!. My staples are: tofu stir-fries, tofu wraps, smoothies, and what I call my "five-minute meals":

- 1 scoop plant protein powder +
- 1 of peanut butter/dry roasted edamame/oats +
- 1 of kale/spinach/broccoli/and/or fruit

This may sound bland, but I enjoy the taste of all of these meals. All are also clean and macro'd properly. The only ingredients I do not necessarily enjoy the taste of are kale and spinach. When I eat them plain, I simply crumple the leaves as small as possible, shove them in my mouth, chew (without attempting to taste) until completely "digested", and wash them down with water. Somehow this is too unbearable for people, yet downing a shot of whiskey or vodka is not. The irony of this is: the former is the king of nutrition, the latter is straight up poison.

If I put them in a smoothie, the taste is completely hidden by the fruit, peanut butter, and protein powder.

Batch Cooking And Storage

Also known as "bulk cooking". Pick a day (or 2) during the week. Or perhaps a day every other week. Create or cook up ingredients (or even entire meals) and store them in the fridge or freezer. As I stated earlier, I do this with wraps. I also do this on a day to day basis, but on a smaller scale:

- Cook up a tofu stir-fry (2 servings) → either:
  - eat one serving and pack the other in a container or thermos

    or
  - pack *both* to bring with me, and eat something simple while, or before I am cooking up the stir-fry itself (I do this all the time—3 meals in under 25 minutes)
- Whip up a massive smoothie, split into 2 or 3 large cups, drink one, pack the other(s). If a fridge is available where I am going, I store in the fridge. If not, I either bring a small cooler, or use a thermos. Bringing a cooler should not turn you off from this concept. This is a small "sacrifice" to pay in order to achieve your body goals and great health.
- My 5-minute meal prep ... I bring:
  - 2 shaker cups with me, each containing a scoop of plant protein powder,
  - one of: dry roasted edamame, peanut butter, or almonds (nuts),
  - and a small plastic bin of baby kale and/or spinach.
  - I also bring either a jug of water, or a few bottles of water.
  - Every 3 hours (starting after my last meal at home), I will:
    - eat a handful (or two) of kale or spinach,
    - eat my desired serving of carbs or fat,
    - and finally, add water to my shaker cup, shake it up, and drink my protein shake. This option takes literally minutes to (both) prepare *and* consume!

I also mentioned coolers, containers, thermos-style containers, and shaker cups. **Keep in mind that these storage devices can also function as portion control.** Whether you intend to or not, over time you will be able to visualize what certain portions look like— especially in respect to the container(s) they are stored in.

The Five-Minute Diet

I have mentioned my "five-minute meals" a number of times up to this point. I want to quickly discuss the ideology behind these meals so you can come up with your own variations.

Protein Powder

Each meal contains plant protein powder at the head. As we have discussed, protein powder is a very quick and convenient option. It takes just *seconds* to mix the powder with water. This can occur by stirring in an uncovered glass/cup, or shaking in a covered cup/water bottle. Once prepared, chug the concoction as protein powder and water is not exactly a treat. However, it is more than bearable.

Raw Greens

Raw greens take even less preparation than protein powder. Take them out of the fridge, rinse with water, and eat or store them. If using broccoli, there is obviously the extra step of cutting off the base. This also only takes a few seconds.

Leafy greens are often available in pre-washed plastic tubs or bags. You can simply pack the tub or bag in a small cooler and bring it with you. Eat a handful and chew until completely digested in your mouth. Do not think about tasting the food! When ready, wash it down with water. Repeat this as desired.

The Carb or Fat Source

The carb and fat source can be a bit more tricky. You need to use sources that take only a few minutes (tops) to prepare. The ingredient list should be "just the food source" or as short as possible! Here are a few examples of potential carb or fat sources.

Carb Source	Fat Source
Dry Roasted Edamame	Nuts & Seeds
Dry Roasted Chickpeas	Nut Butters & Seed Butters
Rice Cakes	Extra Virgin Coconut Oil
Canned Beans	Dark Chocolate (>80%)
Quick Cooking GF Oats	Avocados

5 Cheat Meals And Diet Strictness

Both of these topics have been discussed marginally in prior chapters. I would like to go into a bit more detail to avoid any potential confusion on the subjects. Hearing (reading) the same thing twice also never hurts. While this diet is very simple and straight-forward, I do understand that all of this information can be a bit overwhelming.

Redefining The Cheat Meal

Not all cheat meals are created equally. This should be common sense. Saying this, I have seen *so* many falter in this area of dieting. I want to make it clear: a bad enough cheat meal can erase *days* of perfect eating. This can lead to frustration and regret, which can then lead to falling off completely. Do not let this happen to you!

I will not get into the "how often" side of this just yet. First, let's address the cheat meal itself. What makes a good cheat meal? What are the guidelines? What is considered "over the top"? What exactly constitutes as a cheat meal in the first place?

Cheating is not limited to "too much food in one sitting" and/or consuming non-compliant ingredients. Cheating can also refer to eating too soon (3-hour rule) and/or eating an otherwise healthy meal that isn't macro'd properly (ratio and amount of protein, fats, carbs, etc). Waiting too long to eat can also be considered a cheat, especially if your goal involves putting on some sort of muscle. Keep all of this in mind!

A good cheat meal is not far off from a regular, compliant meal. The macro-nutrient minimums still need to be fulfilled! This is rule number one. The calories, however, can be exceeded. If your normal meals are ~400 calories, a good cheat meal can be up to 600-700 calories—as long as the ingredients are mostly compliant. By this I mean an excess of clean ingredients, with perhaps a small amount of agave (a cheat ingredient) mixed in (for example). Still try to get a green in! But again, this is a cheat meal. If you miss the green, you miss the green.

Here is an example of one of my go-to cheat meals:

Thai Curry Tofu Stir Fry (makes 3-4 servings) - ~ 30 minutes
-1 Package Tofu (~400 calories, ~40g protein) … seasoned with Garlic Powder/Black Pepper
-1 tbsp Extra Virgin Olive Oil (~120 calories, 1 serving of fat)
-1 can Thai Coconut Milk (**700 Calories, 5 servings of fat, ~5g protein**)
-1.5 tbsp Red or Green Curry Paste (~23 calories)
-Decent amount of Broccoli (~50+ calories, ~5g protein)
-1 tsp agave (20 calories, ~5g of sugar) – optional and unnecessary
-300 calories worth of gluten-free pasta or long-grain rice (~1.5-2 servings worth of carbs, 8g protein)
-Basil (for sauce)

Per Serving (3 servings): ~533 calories, 19g protein, 2 servings of fat, ~½ serving of carbs, *tiny* amount of sugar (from the agave)

This is what a smart cheat meal looks like. The ingredients are clean … the macro's are hit … the calories are an excess, but not "over the top"... it contains a green … the sauce perhaps sweetened with agave (or coconut sugar), but a minimal amount … and best of all, it tastes flat out awesome.

Very quickly, this is how you make it:
1. Large Pan: Fry (cubed) tofu in olive oil with garlic powder and black pepper. Flip a few times to evenly cook. Mix in broccoli after ~a flip or two of tofu. Keep broccoli on top of tofu to avoid charring.
2. Small Pan: Mix canned Thai Coconut Milk, Curry Paste, Agave (opt.), and Basil (opt.) → Bring to a boil and then simmer on med-low heat until thickens (this takes at least 10-15 minutes). Stir often.
3. Small to Medium Pot: Boil water, cook pasta or rice until tender/absorbed. Drain and either mix in with stir fry, or keep plain and pour completed stir fry on-top (on each plate).
4. Before the latter part of step 3, combine the sauce from the small pan into everything (tofu & broccoli) that is in the large pan. Stir and cook on low for a few minutes (if need be).

Note: you can also add an onion to this recipe, as well as other vegetables. Do your thing!

What does an awful cheat meal look like? I won't go into specifics, but:

- ignored calorie counts completely (in excess of 600-700)
- ignored macro-nutrient amounts and ratios
- loaded with non-compliant ingredients (sugar, yeast, alcohol, etc)
- eaten within ~an hour or two of prior meal

Compromising For Long-term Success

As I have stated several times in this book, your diet must be consistently strict if you want to achieve a legitimately, low body-fat percentage. By legitimately I mean: cut, ripped, toned, aka extremely confident in your bathing suit. I do not mean simply: "not overweight". This does not equate to confidence! And I don't say this to sound offensive, I am just being completely up-front and honest. Do you really want to learn about a diet-plan that is ineffective?!

Saying this, I want to address another aspect of cheating smart. To be more specific, the timing of cheat meals. This section will be very straightforward and to-the-point.

There are essentially three forms of dieting: cutting, bulking, and somewhere in-between. I went over this in Chapter 3. During cutting, the primary goal is lowering body-fat. This isn't to say it ignores gaining/maintaining muscle (because it doesn't), but again, lowering body-fat is the primary goal. During this time, cheat meals need to be kept to an absolute minimum. In reality, they should not even exist, as (again) even just one cheat meal can erase *days* of perfect eating. If cutting is your goal, you need to be honest with yourself. Literally tell yourself, "no cheat meals"!

Fortunately, legitimate "cutting" is a form of short term dieting. The "in-between portion" of dieting is where most should be at a majority of the time. This stage still prioritizes lowering body-fat and gaining lean muscle, however extremes are not taken (in either direction) to help quicken the process.

Cheating during this phase should still be kept to a minimum, however, it certainly can (and will) occur. You need to have a legitimate idea of how much you can cheat and still remain in this phase (and not accidentally join the bulking club).

Perhaps start at a rate of twice per week. Ask yourself: "Am I making progress towards my goals?" Yes? Great, stick with that. No? Go down to once per week.

If you are miserable and your diet feels too bland? *OK*, try three per week—just know that this *will* hamper your goals. You are relying too much on food for pleasure and comfort! This is when food becomes a drug! I cannot make this any clearer. Food is fuel for survival. The only animal on the planet that purposely relies on food for pleasure is humans.

There are, however, some tricks you can apply to overcome cheat meals. Okay I lied—they aren't tricks. It's called working out. Legitimately working out (not walking or jogging around the neighborhood). Calisthenics, weights—*resistance* exercise (not to mention HIIT work and *grueling* cardio). Give your muscles a reason to grow and your metabolism will rise. Your hormones will optimize. You will be able to consume **more** food.

The closer to exercise you consume cheat meals, the less chance they will have to cause excess body-fat. It really is this simple. And by this I do not mean "consume a cheat meal five minutes before exercise". I mean perhaps the same day. Or an hour before. Or right after. You get the point. Again, the more you workout, the more you can cheat.

What about bulking? Well, this depends on the person and his or her goals. If the goal is maximization of muscle mass over everything else, go ahead and consume a cheat meal every day. Just keep in mind that this will cause an increase in body-fat. Bulking implies that an increase in body-fat is not a deal-breaker. **Create your standard and stick with it.**

6 Supplementation

Supplementation is a hot topic in regards to Vegan eating. I want to spend a bit of time going over a number of popular choices. Keep in mind that many supplements that may appear to be vegan, are not actually vegan (e.g., amino-acids derived from animal sources). Also, realize that essentially "anything and everything" is available in supplement form in today's world. It's a billion dollar industry.

Plant Protein Powder

I have already gone over the uses and perks of using protein powder. I will shift the focus onto actually purchasing this supplement.

There are countless variations of plant protein powders: brown rice protein, pea (gemma) protein, hemp protein, soy protein, potato protein, artichoke protein, quinoa protein, amaranth protein, pumpkin protein, cranberry protein, even alfalfa protein. The majority of protein supplements are a combination of 2-4 of these powders. The primary reason is that each contains different amounts and proportions of essential amino-acids.

Companies will look to "create" an amino-acid profile that mocks a more complete variation, such as whey (whey is the leaner of the two proteins deriving from milk—the other being casein). This is to give assurance to the user (consumer) that the protein he or she is using is optimal for muscle growth and maintenance.

The most popular combinations contain one of rice protein or pea protein (often, both). Neither of these alone is considered a complete protein (containing "sufficient" amounts of the 9 essential amino-acids in adequate proportions). They are combined to boost this amino-acid profile. Companies will boast the "completeness" of the amino-acid profile from the said combination.

On a personal level, I *do* look for a combination, however I do not care as much exactly what the combination is. As long as I see ~20g per 100-120 calories, and the taste and price is right, I am on board. There is no real point in buying (say) rice or pea protein alone, as the combinations are out there.

I just mentioned the amount of protein, the taste, and the price. These are all important for obvious reasons:

1. You want a lean source. 20 grams to 100-120 calories is extremely lean.
2. Taste is vital. Powders are often used to increase the taste of green smoothies. They are also mixed with water (or almond, cashew, soy, etc, milk), in which a poor tasting protein may be overpowering.
3. Value! There are some extremely overpriced companies out there. Do not let the marketing fool you. Multiply grams of protein by the servings, and divide that number by the price to see how much you are paying. For example:

60 servings x 20 grams of protein = 1200grams / $50 = **$1 per 24g** (this would be a decent price, especially for a plant-based protein)

vs

19 servings x 30 grams of protein = 570grams / $44 = **1$ per 13g** (these are the numbers from an extremely popular plant protein that will go unnamed)

Protein powders usually contain at least one sweetener (not all, but most). Fortunately, companies that manufacture plant proteins seem to understand that their target market is very selective when it comes to these sweeteners. I have yet to come across a plant protein that uses artificial sweeteners or straight-up sugar (in its worst forms: "cane sugar", "cane juice", etc).

Typically, you will see a combination of: stevia/steviol, fructose, "natural" vanilla or chocolate flavor, among others. I would not be concerned with any of these, unless of course you have an allergy to stevia (for example). The fructose amount is extremely low when used in protein powders. It will always be towards the end of the ingredient list and the nutrition facts will only show about a gram of sugar per scoop.

Most powders also contain a thickening agent such as guar gum or xanthum gum. Again, these are always going to be in small amounts, and are otherwise harmless (outside of an allergy). If you do not recognize an ingredient, research it on the internet.

This pretty much covers protein powders. As I stated in Chapter 3, I consider it illogical to not use them on a Vegan diet. (lean, time-saving, versatile, taste-boosting, among others)

Vitamin B-12

Most of the information out there states that Vegans must supplement Vitamin B-12, as it is not present in natural plant sources. The body does not need much, but it does need it. Low B-12 levels can lead to various health issues (nervous system, etc—stuff you do not want to mess with). While various Vegan foods are fortified with B-12 (nut milks, soy milks, etc), I recommend using a standalone sub-lingual B-12 supplement. Sub-lingual refers to the dissolving of a tablet or liquid under your tongue. B-12 is not absorbed in high amounts when eaten normally. Therefore, companies started to develop sub-lingual versions.

There is also no harm in consuming too much. This doesn't mean melt 15 tabs under your tongue—I just mean do not get too caught up in the numbers (micrograms, etc). Try to remember to take at least 1 per day. If you miss a day, you will be fine. Issues usually arise from long-term deficiencies.

Again, do not be fooled by marketing. Find a cheap variation from an otherwise reputable company. There are often deals online for buy-one-get-one-half-off 250 tabs for $8 (500 for $12). You will also see ranges of $3 for 60 tabs, to upwards of $20 for the same number of tabs (at a higher microgram # per tab)! Again, the body only needs a small amount, do not get caught up in the micrograms. I usually take 1 a day (2 max, spread out) and prefer to use Methylcobalamin ("Methyl B-12") over the Cyanocobalamin alternative. It is considered the superior form (absorption, etc). Is it really? Who knows—the prices are pretty much the same, so I go for it. If you are at the store and only see Cyanocobalamin, just buy it (and perhaps buy the Methylcobalamin in the future).

I also want to state that the "energy gain" from supplementing with B-12 is not similar to that of a stimulant (such as caffeine). It is one of the situations where a deficiency can cause a decrease in energy (aka, abnormal levels).

So again, do not take multiple in an attempt to "chase a buzz" – it will not work. B-12 will only provide a quick, noticeable energy gain when injected into the muscle. I know this because I have personally taken them. I had low B-12 levels during my meat-eating days (ironically) and was prescribed injections. Please realize that I am not pushing B-12 injections. I am just stating that this is the only form that provides a noticeable energy increase (so you don't bother taking too many tablets).

Vitamin D-3

Vegans pretty much have to supplement Vitamin D-3. The only exception would be individuals that work outside, and in areas that receive a fair amount of sun. When the skin receives sunlight, Vitamin D is produced. Keep in mind that those with naturally darker skin-tones do not absorb as much sunlight as those with lighter skin-tones (therefore produce less Vitamin D). These individuals absolutely should supplement D-3.

Vitamin D-3 is not the same as Vitamin D-2. D-3 is the version we find in fortified foods and supplements. Vitamin D-3 supplements are often created from animal sources and therefore are not Vegan. If it doesn't state "Vegan" somewhere, it isn't. Just as if a product doesn't state "organic" or "gluten free", it probably isn't either. These are labels that only increase the value of product—they will never be purposely suppressed.

These three supplements above should be staples for all Vegans. The rest that I am about to go over are far less important.

Multivitamins

The multivitamin craze has waned quite a bit. I will keep this one short. A multivitamin will not replace the nutrition of a proper diet. I can think of one reason to take one: if you know that for a certain period of time (be it a day, a week, a vacation—whatever) you will not be able to eat greens, veggies, and/or fruits.

For example: You are living on edamame, peanut butter, protein powder and no greens. Perhaps a multivitamin will not hurt here.

"Greens" Powders

Greens powders are essentially the protein powder version of greens. They even come in multivitamin variations (to tie into our last supplement). Examples include: wheatgrass powder, alfalfa powder, spirulina, chlorella, spinach, broccoli, massive combinations of the like, "anti-oxidant blends", probiotics, and anything/everything you can imagine. Some even have caffeine. I view these similarly to how I view multivitamins, just a bit more "natural" and closer to actual food. If you know that for a period of time you will not be able to eat greens, veggies, and fruits, these may be an option. However, they can be pricey and usually taste very poor. I have tried a number of these over the years. I never finish the container/package and usually end up wasting my money.

Creatine

This one is for the weightlifting crowd. Yes, there is "Vegan creatine" out there. How it is sourced or created, I do not know—but it does exist. Cranberries do contain small amounts of creatine, however I would assume that Vegan creatine is synthetically derived/created.

Anyone who has ever taken creatine knows what it does, and what it claims to do. First, I will hit the claims. Creatine claims to increase muscle size, strength, and even cognitive function (brain function). I am not sure how the third was studied, but lets address the first two.

Yes, creatine will put on a few pounds of mass—mostly in the form of water. After just a few days of usage, your muscles will appear "bigger". This is non-disputable. The idea is that your muscles already contain creatine, but not necessarily the maximal amount. So by supplementing it, you are saturating (maxing out) the levels. The end goal is increased maximal strength, and strength endurance.

Does it increase strength? Studies claim that it does—marginally. I have seen numbers such as 3% and 5%. 3% and 5% *are* actually large numbers, especially for those in sports such as power lifting, strongman competitions, football, and the like.

What is my take on creatine? Quite frankly it sketches me out. I took it on and off for a few years in my early 20s. It just seems so unnatural. You take this tiny bit of powder for just a few days and your body visibly changes. Not in the way that steroids change it— but again, the change is indeed noticeable (especially for those who track their physiques almost religiously). Stop taking it, and the body will return to normal.

A quick internet search will reveal several contradicting studies. Some say it is *only* beneficial and harmless. Others link it to cancer (yikes). Then again, there are contradicting studies for pretty much everything.

Why did I stop? Well, I am not a competitive power-lifter or strongman. I don't care about the potential edge. Those cancer studies scare the you-know-what out of me. Even if the risk is 1% – I wouldn't take that risk for even a 10% strength increase (let alone 3%)—that's just me.

Not to mention, all of my max lifts took place off of creatine. And my best physique was off creatine. This isn't to say these things wouldn't have improved if I took creatine *at that time*. But I got there without it.

If you do decide to try it, be sure to drink a ton of water. Creatine is dehydrating by nature. Also be sure to research the dosages. Modern studies claim that far less is required for muscle saturation than previously thought. I am talking dosages as low a ~2.5 grams/day versus what individuals used to do: take upwards of 20g a day for a few days, then 5g a day to maintain. I find anything over 5g to be completely absurd. Please do the research.

BCAAs (Branched Chain Amino-acids)

Another one for the weightlifting crowd … I will keep this one short. First, I must mention again that most sources of "BCAAs" are not vegan. The vegan sources are few and far between.

What are BCAAs? Three amino-acids: Leucine, Isoleucine, and Valine. I am not going to get into the role of each—but generally speaking, these three are said to aid in muscle recovery, growth, and endurance. Supplement companies dose them in specific proportions, usually a 2-1-1 ratio (e.g., 3500mg Leucine, 1750mg Isoleucine, 1750mg Valine). They are often put in "intraworkout" supplements, as well as both pre and post-workout supplements.

These amino-acids are already present in protein powders and everyday foods. The individual that uses BCAAs is someone that feels the need to add even more amino-acids to his or her diet for whatever reason (strength, recovery, etc). Generally speaking, they are not necessary.

Probiotics

Probiotics are said to aid in digestion and maintenance of a healthy gut ("beneficial bacteria"). I cannot help, but call "BS" on this one. I have used them in the past, and each time it resulted in acne and stomach issues. I feel like this is one of those quick fixes for individuals that have digestion issues from a poor diet. Just fix the diet!

The laughable part to me is how much yogurt is pushed due to its "natural" probiotics. Yogurt itself is straight-up casein—the protein in milk that humans have issues digesting in the first place.

As I stated in Chapter 2, the only reason I can see using a probiotic is during and/or after using an antibiotic. And even then, I'd much prefer my body to naturally fix itself on its own. This whole probiotic and fermented food craze is nothing but a craze … a money-grab (in my opinion). I say this because I have tried all of these crazes. I have experimented so much with diet in my lifetime.

I group probiotics and fermented foods with yeast—and you already know yeast is a massive "no-no" on this diet. If you want a healthy gut, simply follow this diet. Eat Vegan and do not consume sugar, yeast, and gluten. Do not bother with probiotics and fermented foods.

I promise you this: if you go two weeks with ZERO: meat, dairy, sugar, yeast, gluten, fermented foods, probiotics, and overly processed foods, your skin will clear and you will not get a stomach ache during this time. The only way to get a stomach ache while following these guidelines (to a T) is through some sort of drug (too much caffeine, for example).

Electrolyte Powders

Popular sports drinks boast their electrolytes. Electrolytes are a marketer's dream, simply because how cool the word sounds. How about potassium? Or sodium? Or calcium? Bicarbonate? Chloride? Magnesium? Phosphate? Do these sound familiar? Because these are all electrolytes. Sports drinks and electrolyte powders replenish a combination of these electrolytes. The issue with sports drinks is they also add about 34 grams of sugar to the concoction to make it taste good. Not to mention the multiple color dyes to make it look exotic.

Electrolyte powders are a great substitute for traditional sports drinks as they (the good ones) contain just the electrolytes and often a better sweetener choice, such as stevia. Electrolytes are sweated out during intense exercise. They are commonly used by endurance athletes (runners, cyclists, and the like).

7 Traveling And Eating Out

Situations are going to arise when adhering to this diet becomes a bit more complicated. Fortunately, there are strategies and techniques that will at least dampen potential damage done during this span. I urge you to go easy on yourself in these situations—do not go "all in" or "all out". A <u>mix</u> of compliance and cheating will allow you to quickly erase any setbacks that may occur (when you are back on your normal schedule). Attempting to be 100% perfect will cause a high amount of stress when circumstances arise that are not in your control. This can ruin an otherwise enjoyable experience for both yourself, and those around you. On the flip-side, eating "anything and everything" can and will obliterate prior **weeks** of progress.

Traveling

The amount of preparation you put in before travel will determine how compliant (to the diet) you will remain throughout your trip. Obviously, packing your fridge is not an option. There are, however, certain foods and supplements that I consider staples to bring along when traveling.

<u>**Protein Powder:**</u> This is an obvious one. I will not say much here, but know that you do not have to pack an entire 5lb container. Multiply the days you are gone by 2 or 3 scoops of protein. If you want to pack more, go for it. If you *do* want to pack an entire container (and it fits), more power to you.

I also recommend packing "shaker cups" if you have them. Or really, anything that can be shaken to mix the powder with water. A funnel and water bottle works just as well. If you do use shaker cups, try to rinse them with warm water and soap in-between use.

<u>**Nuts, Seeds, or a Nut Butter:**</u> This is your fat option. All are extremely convenient for traveling. (See the Fat column on the food list for specific options.) Nuts and seeds work great for carry-on. Coconut oil is another option here as well and can double as a mild form of sun-tan oil (approximately an SPF of 4, so not very strong).

Dry Roasted Edamame: Dry roasted edamame (young soybeans) is a great option for convenient carbohydrates. Not only is edamame a complete protein, it is minimally processed and requires zero preparation. If you are not a fan of soy, perhaps try dry-roasted chickpeas.

A "Greens Powder" or Multivitamin: If you know that (relatively) healthy food is going to be hard to come by, perhaps purchase a "greens powder" or multivitamin to bring along with you. This is just to get *something* with vitamins in your system.

Protein Bars: While protein bars are not the best option for a regular diet (at least not too often), they can be an absolute godsend when traveling. Look for the plant-based bar that contains the highest grams of protein. There are bars out there that are around ~300 calories and contain 20+ grams of protein. These are a better option than higher calories/lower protein bars that contain mostly complex carbohydrates (oats) and peanut butter. Remember the numbers we went over in Chapter 3: ~350-400+ calories, 20+ grams of protein per meal. If I know I will have little control over my environment, I will pack literally an entire box (or two) of protein bars.

There isn't much else to mention here that we haven't already gone over in Chapter 3. I do recommend setting your alarm for every 3 hours (or some sort of reminder) so you at least have a rough idea of when you should be eating.

Eating Out

A large part of traveling is going out to eat. This section will cover eating at restaurants both while traveling, and while at home. Before I get into menus and options, I want to make one thing clear: if your goal is to lose body-fat, you should try not to eat out too often. Try to be in direct control of your meal creation and preparation, as often as possible. This way:

- you know the exact ingredients and their amounts/proportions
- you know the exact quality of the ingredients

- you know how the ingredients are being cooked or prepared

Saying this, I will first address eating at Vegan restaurants. Vegan restaurants are a gift to Vegans. They aren't exactly on every street corner. If you encounter one, I encourage you to bend the rules. Try the fake meat ... the quesadilla ... the mock burger. This is one of the few times I consider it acceptable to eat for pleasure.

This is purely a once-in-a-while thing. This doesn't mean every week! Remember, the more you eat out, the more body-fat you will have. It's a very straight-forward concept.

What about non-Vegan restaurants? Well, it depends on where you are going:

(note: I am referring to restaurants in America)

Chinese Food: Chinese food can be tricky because of sauces and butters. Does that Sesame Tofu dish contain an animal product? Do any dishes contain chicken broth? Whether you ask, or simply trust the chef is your call. Assuming the dishes are Vegan, they are still all going to be extremely caloric and sugary. The option is always available to split the dish into two portions—remember that.

Many Chinese restaurants have a tofu dish. If they do not, you will probably end up with some sort of vegetable fried rice, or other vegetable based dish. Definitely opt for the sauce on the side (if you choose to eat it) and just use a tiny bit. The sauce is loaded with ingredients that will directly cause body-fat—I can't say it any clearer.

If you are concerned about not receiving enough protein from a tofu-less dish, simply bring a small protein drink with you (perhaps in a shaker cup). If you are worried about bringing it inside, consume it immediately before or after.

You can use this trick for any restaurant that does not offer a plant-based protein source. Scour the menu for: a plant-based carbohydrate or fat, a salad or roasted/raw vegetables, and complete the meal with a protein shake (water with protein powder).

Italian Food: For former meat eaters, this one is depressing. Italian restaurants are very limited in terms of Vegan dishes. I am not even talking about relatively healthy dishes. The options are just so few and far between. I would do the protein drink trick along with a salad or perhaps some pasta in tomato sauce (and tell the chef "no meat sauce", etc). Do not load up on bread (as tempting as it is)!

Japanese Food: Japanese restaurants always have vegetable sushi: Cucumber rolls, cucumber avocado, sweet potato, etc. Again, you can go this route and combine with a protein drink before/during/or after. Some restaurants have a tofu or bean curd dish, as well as mixed vegetable dishes. I usually go the roll route, however.

Indian Food: Indian restaurants are always loaded with vegetarian options. With this comes plenty of Vegan variations/options as well. I would ask the waiter for recommendations on dishes.

Thai Food: Thai restaurants are usually loaded with unique Tofu dishes. Often with an insanely good curry sauce (coconut milk, etc), vegetables, and a side of rice. Just eat the whole thing (unless it is enormous, then split into two portions).

Mexican/Columbian Food: Beans, rice, vegetables and all their variations. Guacamole, salsa, tortillas, etc. Make sure you let the waiter/waitress know "no cheese/dairy".

Mediterranean and Middle Eastern: Hummus (chickpeas), olive oil, vegetables, veggie wraps/flat-breads/gyros/pita (will contain wheat/gluten, ask about egg), tabbouleh, baba ganoush, falafel, among others.

There is not much else to say in regards to eating out that isn't already common sense. Just remember everything from Chapter 3 about macro-ing (protein, carbs, fats) and portion sizes. Again, do not be afraid to eat half, and save the rest for ~3 hours later!

I do use the protein powder trick often. I sometimes use a protein bar instead—especially if I know I will be getting something small and light (and relatively low in protein), such as a salad. I encourage you to obsess over macro-nutrients. This will change the way you view meals and directly result in healthier eating.

My final piece of advice here is: opt for a water as your beverage. Eating out already constitutes as a cheat meal. Do not make it any worse by consuming 400 calories worth of soda. There needs to be a compromise somewhere.

8 Exercise And Mental Preparation

I have brought up physical exercise in several chapters. Exercise is *extremely* important for the body and mind. Humans seem to forget that they are (also) animals at the most convenient of times. Primarily, these times are eating and exercise. Obviously the majority of this book has been dedicated to the eating—now I will address exercise.

My Recommendations

Exercise can come in various forms. Some are extremely effective, while many are not. I am going to list a variety of exercise types that I know have the potential to produce awesome results. Not just for muscle and body-fat, but the body and mind as a whole.

Body-weight Exercise

Body-weight exercise usually refers to forms of calisthenics, gymnastics, and human movement. Every single person on this planet should be doing some form of body-weight exercise. Proper human (ape) movements are corrective by nature. What I mean by this is: if you perform certain "natural" movements (from an animal perspective) **correctly**, pain, strength, and mobility will improve. The issue with this is the "western lifestyle" has taken humans so far away from this, that attempting to get back into it is extremely difficult. **The movements are no longer natural and *need to be re-learned properly.*** I cannot stress this enough. Improper body-weight (yes, even body-weight) movements *will* cause damage to the body. This potential damage can increase exponentially when combined with "high rep" variations.

What can you do about this? Well, luckily we live in a time when information is just a few clicks away. Just please realize that anyone can post information onto the web. **There is just as much misinformation out there, as there is quality information.** And if a viewer is uninformed about a topic, he or she will have a rough time discerning between the two.

I urge you to check the individual's (who posted the information) credentials. Right now we are talking about body-weight exercise. For this topic, look into high level (Olympic) gymnasts. Gymnasts are the masters of body-weight movement and are the strongest athletes on the planet. Especially when it comes to the upper body, core, and body control.

If the body-weight exercise is sprinting (for example), find information from an Olympic-level sprinter or coach (or at least "NCAA Division-1"). Long distance running, find a professional marathoner. My point is this: there is so much information out there. If you look hard enough, you *will* find high level sources. These same concepts apply to anything and everything you can think of.

Lifting Weights
This is the topic with the most misinformation out there on a wide scale. I will keep this very simple. Do not listen to the individual based solely on his or her physique. Physique is 95% diet. By this, I do not mean diet alone will build muscle. I mean a good diet combined with even sub-optimal exercise (poor form, using machines, etc) and programming (the exercise plan itself) can still lead to an impressive physique.

If you want to learn how to lift, find the best power-lifters in the world, and study their technique. Power-lifting is not to be confused with bodybuilding. Power-lifting refers to the actually lifts themselves. Mainly the big three lifts (deadlift, squat, benchpress), but also the "accessory work" (isolating triceps, etc). Bodybuilding simply refers to "getting on stage and showing off your body". How that body is created can vary massively.

To be more specific about misinformation in this realm, there are certain routines (that are otherwise not-so-great) that have spread like wildfire over the years, simply because the person promoting it had an impressive physique. I will get to the routine in a minute, but I also want to state that the **original sources** of these routines are (strictly) bodybuilders that take (took) steroids and pro-hormones (and whose goals are primarily "aesthetics", *not* functionality).

This isn't to say that these routines cannot still build a ton of muscle (they will). The issue is the *way* they build this muscle. And the lack of attention to detail in regard to technique. Again, get the technique from a high-level power-lifter, not a bodybuilder.

The routine I speak of is the: "chest day", "arm day", "leg day", "shoulder day", "back day", etc, routine. The chest day usually has ~two types of free weight presses, perhaps a machine press or two, a few sets of "flys", among others. "Back day" will have a few variations of free weight rows, perhaps a row machine or two, some "lat pull-downs", and potentially the individual will attempt to throw in an actual pull-up. The issue with these types of routines is not always the exercises themselves. The issue is that:

1. these routines *completely* fatigue individual muscle groups for *days*.. this is not ideal for sports/competition
2. these routines do not prioritize technique and full body lifts
3. these routines use a ton of isolation exercises
4. these routines often include *way* too much machine usage

If you do choose to follow these types of routines: spend the majority of time on the big lifts, limit machine usage, and hybrid the routine with gymnastics and/or power-lifting principles.

Cardio

There are several different forms of cardio. The difference is mainly how each taxes the body. Is it high intensity for a short duration (HIIT, for example)? Is it low intensity for a long duration (long distance running, for example)? Or is it high intensity for a high duration (certain sports and forms of circuit training)?

The variety that has gained the most popularity in recent years is HIIT—High Intensity Interval Training. (I am not saying this is the form you must do, I just know the other two are pretty much common knowledge—for most). HIIT refers to a short period of high intensity exercise (to raise your heart rate), immediately followed by a short rest (to let your heart rate come back down), only to raise the intensity again and repeat this pattern. Often, participants wear heart-rate monitors to keep track of when to start, and when to rest. Set-time intervals are also common practice.

Everyone should perform at least some form of cardio. The choice can be goal dependent, or simply whichever variation is preferred.

Sports And Martial Arts

Sports and martial arts can also be very effective forms of exercise. This of course, depends on the activity and your intensity level. There are several perks to taking part in sports and martial arts. The first is obviously the objective of learning a skill. How useful the skill is, again, depends on the activity choice. The second is the potential of an adrenaline rush and the "fun-factor". This combination can make exercise feel easy. The fatigue (crash) may not even kick in until the activity is over. The third benefit is the social aspect. Sports and martial arts are great for making friends and meeting new people. Socializing is an important aspect of life.

How Often

This depends on the type of activity, your goal(s), and ultimately the program you are on. I will say this though: you should be challenging your body a minimum of three times per week. By "challenging", I mean putting in high effort and focus, and seeking to improve every single session. Perfect the technique. Increase the weight. Progress to the harder variation (but not till the regressed variation is flawless). This goes for every activity: weights, sports, martial arts, calisthenics, gymnastics—everything. **Do not just "go through the motions".**

Exercise is also great for the mind and can be a legitimate form of meditation. If you are breathing, moving, and focusing on a goal within an activity, chances are you are not thinking about:
- your job
- your worries
- your stresses and other potential negative thoughts.

Over time, this will lead to a higher level of clear-headedness and peace of mind.

This brings us to the next part of this chapter: **Mental Preparation**.

Priorities

Everyone is busy—I get it. But **this is your health**! Forget body-image for a minute. Your health has a direct effect on the quality of your life. You can literally lose *decades* by failing to prioritize it! So while I completely understand you have a job to go to, a family to take care of, a social life—I just want to remind you of the **importance of your health!** The entire point of this book is not just teaching you how to eat. It is strategies to incorporate healthy eating into a busy lifestyle. This is why I bring up ideas like the five-minute meals. I want this diet to be EASY! Is peanut butter, protein powder, and a handful of spinach the "holy grail" of meals? Of course not! But is it better than 99.9% of the meals the average person puts in his or her body? I'd make that bet in a heartbeat.

So again, I understand you have other priorities. I am not saying drop them all and jump on this diet. I am saying, put them in order of true importance. Put diet towards the top of the list. Not above family, but perhaps right under it. I would even argue that it is more important than your job. If your job is negatively affecting your health, perhaps you should start applying to new ones. You live one life and you die—this is our reality as humans. Not to sound grim, but why sugarcoat it?

Getting back to body image for a minute ... I *do* think it's important. Obviously what other people think about your body is "none of your business" (aka it shouldn't matter or upset you) – but the other end of the spectrum (you *truly* loving your body) can bring about so much good. The confidence, the peace of mind, the potential to be a positive role model. The potential to have people ask you, "Hey, you look great ... what do you eat?". You let them know you are a Vegan and BAM—just like that you potentially influenced another individual to go Vegan! How would that make you feel? How many animals' lives could this save? How awesome would this be for the environment ... for another human being to go Vegan? This is the way you should be thinking! If you truly believe in Veganism, simply being a positive, kind, upbeat, healthy and in-shape Vegan is the absolute #1 way to spread it. Nothing else comes close. Not picketing, not yelling at meat-eaters, not even getting people to watch those disturbing documentaries.

The Pleasure Principle

In Freud's *Project for a Scientific Psychology (1895)*, he came up with a theory termed "the pleasure principle". He claimed that pain and pleasure are the basis for all human behavior ... that humans seek to avoid pain, and experience pleasure. He also stated (and I am paraphrasing) that: maturity is "learning to endure the pain of deferred gratification".

You may have also heard of this concept from "self-help gurus" such as Anthony (Tony) Robbins. Mr. Robbins asks his listeners (and readers) to logically think about the pleasure principle when it comes to decisions in life. More specifically, to think about the potential long-term pain, versus the potential long-term pleasure.

You probably already know where I am going with this. This concept is an awesome tool for dieting. Let's use sugary foods as an example. Sugary foods provide short term pleasure (there is even a dopamine response in the brain during consumption!—the pleasure chemical). However, sugar also leads to body-fat and potentially disease (long-term pain). *Seconds* of pleasure that can lead to days, weeks, months, and years of emotional and/or physical pain. The choice here should be obvious.

Mental Clarity

The final concept we will cover is mental clarity aka "thinking clearly". If you are an individual whose mind is always racing, know that this is a direct reflection of your daily choices—*not* some sort of "focusing disorder". An overactive mind is the result of too much stimulation. If you do choose to believe in focusing disorders, the antidote is the same regardless.

The mind is a computer. The more information it receives, the more likely it is to race. (This can literally cause anxiety.) **The mind cannot distinguish between useful and useless information. It attempts to store everything.** Think about how computers perform that are loaded with programs, music, photos, viruses (negative thoughts) ... processing slows down, errors occur. You get the picture. The good thing is, this is all fixable.

I will give you three methods that will assist in controlling this issue (I am sure there are more). The first is exercise and physical activity. I already went over this one. During physical activity, you breathe often and fully. (When your mind races, your breathing becomes shallow and less frequent.) Proper breathing is <u>vital</u> for optimal brain function—this is a fact, not a theory. Exercise also optimizes hormone levels and "feel-good" chemicals in the brain.

The next method is meditation. Meditation is real. I want to make this clear. All meditation is, is consistently breathing while relaxing your entire body. This takes place in absence of stimulation. No noise, no television, no checking your phone, nothing. For the first "x" amount of minutes, your mind will attempt to race. This may even go on for 30-40 minutes. However, if you stick with it, and just *keep relaxing and breathing*, eventually you will "wake up" to a calm, quiet and serene existence. Your body will be <u>vibrating</u> with feel-good energy. When you begin to actively think again, you will notice that you are now *attacking* problems with potential solutions. Thinking of actions that can be taken to improve a situation. Your mind will be absent of worry and anxiety.

If you have attempted to meditate and failed miserably, I have two recommendations for you. The first is to set a timer and keep trying. First, for just 5 minutes at a time. When this becomes too easy, bump it up to 10 minutes. Again, the goal is just to relax and breathe for the duration during this "practice". Keep increasing the duration little by little over time.

The second recommendation is using a float tank. "Float studios" and "float spas" are starting to pop up all over the place. The float tanks they provide are *vessels* for meditation. A float tank is usually in the shape of a large rectangular water tank or pod. It is much large enough to avoid any potential claustrophobia. The tank contains less than a foot of water. The water is heated to the same temperature as the surface of your skin and filled with roughly a thousand pounds of epsom salt. This concentration of salt allows your body to "float" freely and effortlessly in the water.

During the experience, there is no sound or light (unless you choose to have calm music playing or leave the light on). Trust me—leave it all off (your phone as well). The floating effect *completely* relaxes the body (if you let it!). This takes care of any potential physical tension during an attempted meditation. When you combine this with a complete lack of stimulation, the result is a perfect setting for meditation. As long as you relax and focus on your breath, you will eventually reach what is known as the "meditative state" (that I described a few paragraphs ago).

These tanks are so effective, that they are probably the only manner in which the majority of the population can reach the meditative state. Saying this, I consider them a "must try" in life. It is not exactly cheap for a session (~60-70 bucks per 90 minutes), but it is worth it—at least once or twice, or until you have reached the meditative state. This is too important a concept to go through life ignoring.

The third method I will throw at you (for achieving mental clarity) is a "low-information diet". I am not sure who the originator of this concept is—I got it from an author/entrepreneur named Timothy Ferriss (he may very well be the originator—regardless, he is getting the credit).

The goal of a low-information diet is to modulate all of the information that you put into your brain. Simply put: if the information is not directly important to you achieving your goal(s), block it out. Do not browse the web. Do not watch the news. Do not watch TV. Do not partake in anything that puts information into your mind that you do not need. It's a **full-focus** approach toward smashing your goal(s). Like I said, your brain cannot discern between useful and useless information—it attempts to store it all!

9 Why Go Vegan?

Generally speaking, humans choose to abide by a Vegan lifestyle for (at least) one of three reasons:

- to literally save the lives of hundreds of animals
- to reduce negative impact on the environment/our planet
- and to (potentially) reap the health benefits of a plant-based diet

I am going to break this chapter down into two sections: Health and Morality.

Health

I want to start this section off by mentioning that a **Vegan diet is only as healthy as the food choices that the individual makes on a consistent basis.** Simply cutting out meat, dairy, and eggs does not necessarily equate to "excellent health". It's a good start, but Vegans can still obviously consume most forms of sugar and overly processed foods (and many do). Vegans can also overeat.

There are studies that link dairy and meat (red meat in particular) to diseases such as cancer and heart disease. However, this is not the angle I want to take in this section. Everyone has already heard of these studies—the fact is, studies are not enough to cause change on a massive scale. If studies (alone) were highly effective:

- no one would consume sugar, alcohol, cigarettes, etc
- no one would overeat
- no one would support corporations and ideas that destroy our planet
- everyone would work out a ton

I have mentioned in prior chapters the idea of experimenting with diet plans over a span of one to two weeks (preferably, two). This gives a large enough time-frame to truly see and feel any potential benefits. I want to address both of these notions: seeing results and feeling good.

Seeing results is extremely important (to humans) for obvious reasons. Regardless of what individuals say, everyone wants to at least look to be in-shape. The fact is, we live in a superficial society that values physical looks over pretty much everything. And this isn't limited to human looks. Even animals are treated largely based upon how they look! (Think of how a dog or cat is treated versus a turkey or chicken.)

Seeing results boosts confidence. Confidence boosts mood and a boosted mood results in feeling good. There is a reason that obesity and depression often go hand-in-hand. Fat-gaining foods produce a short term dopamine spike and (obviously) gain fat! This combination is a recipe for depression. Constant dopamine spikes equates to overall lower dopamine levels. This isn't just: "Oh I hate the way I look, now I am upset" – No! These are literally chemicals in the brain that are being altered based off of *food choices*!

When an individual decides to eat "100% clean", the script is flipped:
- no more dopamine spikes → levels normalize
- better body = better mood and mind

I encourage you to test this concept. Go two weeks on this diet with one-hundred percent compliancy. ***One-hundred percent***—*not* "sometimes following the diet", but also:
- eating junk here and there
- drinking too much caffeine
- not drinking enough water
- consuming alcohol
- etc, etc

To truly test a diet, it *needs* to be done with 100% compliancy. (I cannot repeat this enough!) Otherwise the diet is not actually being tested. Other factors are coming into play that are not part of the diet.

Yes, diets take discipline! But in the "western world", we humans already have it so good. Every other animal on the planet (outside of our pets) is forced to fight **every single day** just to *survive*. The idea of comfort is non-existent—let alone *eating for comfort!*

Food is fuel! Relying on it for comfort and pleasure will lead to health issues. Throw out the genetics excuse! Genetics do not cause type 2 diabetes and heart disease. I do not buy this and neither should you! It is completely illogical. Environment and choice trumps genetics 99% of the time. Again, test the diet for two weeks and see for yourself.

I want to address one more topic in regards to health. On the following two pages is a chart that compares the physiology of "natural" carnivores (meat eaters), to herbivores (plant eaters), to omnivores (plant and meat eaters), to humans.

This chart helps explain ideas such as: "why humans cannot consume raw meat, while cats (for example) can". Look at the stomach acidity. Look at the digestive tract.

I am not trying to convince here. I simply feel that a chart like this may help explain why studies link the consumption of animal products to potentially deadly diseases. *Should* humans be consuming meat, dairy, and eggs?

I have mentioned already: most meat eaters that eat otherwise healthy do "just fine". But is it *optimal* (versus eating 100% plant-based)? It's difficult to make this claim. I just know that I feel at least "just as good" eating 100% plant-based. Then again, there is obviously more to feeling good than diet and nutrition alone.

Physical Characteristics Of Animals

	Herbivore	Human	Carnivore	Omnivore
Facial Muscles	Well developed	Well developed	Reduced to allow mouth to gape	Reduced
Jaw Type	Expanded Angle	Expanded Angle	Angle not expanded	Angle not expanded
Jaw Joint Location	Above the plane of the molars	Above the plane of the molars	On same plane as molar teeth	On same plane as molar teeth
Jaw Motion	No shear, good side-to-side, front-to-back	No shear, good side-to-side, front-to-back	Shearing, minimal side-to-side	Shearing, minimal side-to-side
Major Jaw Muscles	Masseter and pterygoids	Masseter and pterygoids	Temporalis	Temporalis
Mouth Opening vs. Head Size	Small	Small	Large	Large
Teeth (Incisors)	Broad, flattened and spade shaped	Broad, flattened and spade shaped	Short and pointed	Short and pointed
Teeth (Canines)	Dull and short or long (for defense) or none	Short and blunted	Long, sharp, and curved	Long, sharp, and curved
Teeth (Molars)	Flattened with cusps vs complex surface	Flattened with nodular cusps	Sharp, jagged, and blade shaped	Sharp blades and/or flattened
Chewing	Extensive Chewing Necessary	Extensive Chewing Necessary	None; swallows food whole	Swallows food whole and/or simple crushing
Saliva	Carbohydrate digesting enzymes	Carbohydrate digesting enzymes	No digestive enzymes	No digestive enzymes
Stomach Type	Simple or multiple chambers	Simple	Simple	Simple

	Herbivore	Human	Carnivore	Omnivore
Stomach Acidity	PH 4 to 5 with food in stomach	PH 4 to 5 with food in stomach	Less than or equal to pH 1 with food in stomach	Less than or equal to pH 1 with food in stomach
Stomach Capacity	Less than 30% of total volume of digestive tract	21% to 27% of total volume of digestive tract	60% to 70% of total volume of digestive tract	60% to 70% of total volume of digestive tract
Length of Small Intestine	10 to more than 12 times body length	10 to 11 times body length	3 to 6 times body length	4 to 6 times body length
Colon	Long, complex; may be sacculated	Long, sacculated	Simple, short, and smooth	Simple, short, and smooth
Liver	Cannot detoxify vitamin A	Cannot detoxify vitamin A	Can detoxify vitamin A	Can detoxify vitamin A
Kidney	Moderately concentrated urine	Moderately concentrated urine	Extremely concentrated urine	Extremely concentrated urine
Nails	Flattened nails or blunt hooves	Flattened nails	Sharp claws	Sharp claws

Source: Mills, Milton R., M.D. " The Comparative Anatomy of Eating." *Vegsource*. Web. 8 June 2017.<http://www.vegsource.com/news/2009/11/the-comparative-anatomy-of-eating.html>.

Morality

I don't think it's a stretch to claim that the majority of Vegan converts did so for moral reasons. To be more particular: the welfare of animals. Yes, going Vegan is arguably the best choice a human can make for the environment as well. But the choice more than likely originated with animals. I am going to throw you a few of my arguments on why I believe that it is immoral to eat and use animal products. My intent here is not to rant or call anyone out. These are simply my views on the topic!

Since the year 2000, over 150 billion (150,000,000,000) land animals have been slaughtered in the United States alone. (~9 billion/year) Chickens, turkeys, pigs, cows, ducks, sheep, and lambs (in order from most to least killed). I am using the US as an example because I reside in the US. I am familiar with the people and the culture(s).

The amount of animals killed in the US is a direct reflection of the market demand: The majority of the population regularly consumes meat → it is legal to operate a slaughterhouse → slaughterhouses sell meat → animals get slaughtered.

Every single time a human purchases meat, the demand to kill an animal rises. This is a fact that ~99% of humans *choose* to ignore.

"I didn't kill the animal … I love animals".

Statements like this is why Vegans go crazy. We watch humans simultaneously treat cats and dogs with love, and at the same time consume meat, dairy, and eggs. **There is absolutely no difference between a chicken, turkey, cow, pig, cat, or dog.** Every single emotion our pet emits, the animal that was tortured and brutally murdered for that steak *also* once emit**ted**.

Our dog or cat is not more intelligent. It does not feel more pain. It does not exhibit more fear. It doesn't want to die any less than that cow, turkey, pig, sheep, duck, or lamb.

No being comes into this planet wanting to die. You try to kill a human, it will run or fight back. You try to kill a wild animal, it will run or fight back. You try to catch a fish, it will swim away. You try to kill even an insect, it will scurry or fly away. **No being wants to die. This is the basis of Veganism—compassion.** Yet somehow Vegans are the ones that are made fun of and considered extreme.

Think again about our pets and the personal connection we have with them. Think about how "human" they actually are. Their distinct personalities. The little quirks that make them unique. Not far off from the traits that make humans unique. Frighteningly similar, actually.

So why do we treat farm animals different? Well, think of how we were raised, and how most of the people around us were raised. *Pretty much the same.* Human behavior derives from what is considered normal and acceptable by the majority of the population (societal norms). The majority of the population has consumed meat since far before any of us showed up. Therefore, most of us do as well, as the trend has yet to be broken. And it's a tricky trend to break because it's big business, and big business literally runs governments.

Big business also specializes in marketing. Look at the commercials: people smiling and laughing while eating meat—never anything about how the meat is sourced. Invoke the emotion of happiness → tie it into eating meat → brainwash the population into thinking "meat is great!"

That's all it is ... extremely effective marketing combined with habit. The goal of marketing is very straight-forward: **increase sales.** Mention the good, hide the bad, make a buck.

As consumers, it is our duty to take a step back and truly investigate the product: "Do I need this product?" ... "What are the 'pros and cons'?" ... "Is this product moral?" ... "Are there similar alternatives?"

These are the questions I asked myself before going Vegan. Just days later I made the switch, as the answers were very one-sided:

- I don't need the product. Sure, it tastes good and is offered (sold) pretty much everywhere. However, plant-based foods also taste extremely good. **They also contain every macro-nutrient and essential amino-acid found in animal products.** And the only micro-nutrient missing (B12) can be supplemented in just seconds per day.

- Obviously the product is immoral. It is probably the most immoral product a consumer can purchase as an innocent being is tortured and killed to create it. And these innocent beings are tortured and killed by the billions.

- There are tons of alternatives. Alternative lean protein sources (tofu, tempeh, plant protein powder, seitan). Alternative saturated fats (coconut oil). Alternative "meat-like" textures (tofu, seitan, textured vegetable protein). Alternative "milks" that are also far healthier (almond milk, cashew milk, rice milk, soy milk, coconut milk).

Think about the societal norms in regards to the treatment of animals. Individuals become outraged over dog and cat abuse, yet those same individuals have no issue enjoying a burger or ham sandwich.

Individuals can spend *years* in prison for abusing a dog, yet (again) 99% of the population is directly responsible for the deaths of hundreds of animals *per person*. None of this makes any sense!

Think about how Vegans are treated and labeled:
- "Extremists"
- "Aggressive"
- "Weirdos"
- "Violent"
- "Abusive"
- "Weak"
- "Pretentious"

This makes even less sense! These are simply people who **do not believe in violence.** And these words are spewed by individuals that *do* directly contribute to murder and violence.

Please hear me out: We have been lied to. We have been misled. Humans do not need to consume animals products. I have been Vegan for **years** and feel awesome. I still have high energy. I still have low body-fat. I am still packing on muscle. I am still increasing my strength in the gym. *Nothing* has changed for the worse!

So I challenge you: Take two weeks to test this diet. *It's just two weeks!* Follow my instructions and experience "the other side". See for yourself that you can and will thrive on a plant-based diet!

My Go-To Recipes

Before I get into specific recipes, I want to quickly review the concepts behind creating your own recipes. It is far more important to understand this, than to memorize actual recipes.

1. Choose food items from the Food List in Chapter 1.
2. Avoid the culprit ingredients from Chapter 2.
3. Follow the meal-building instructions from Chapter 3:
   - If heading a meal with tofu, protein powder, or tempeh (or seitan, if you so choose):
     - Each meal = protein column + carbohydrate OR fat column (or a split) + veggies (greens!)
     - Shoot for 20+ grams of protein from 100-200 calories. 1 serving of fat or 100-200+ calories from complex carbohydrates (beans, rice, sweet potatoes, oats, etc). Greens (spinach, kale, broccoli, etc) or other veggies if greens are not available. The next option is fruit.
   - If heading a meal with a bean (as the protein source):
     - Each Meal = ~200+ calories from beans + very little fat (if any) + greens and veggies
     - A portion of the beans' calories can be substituted for a grain (rice, etc) or sweet potatoes/yams.

Some Common Choices From The Food List

Protein	Carbohydrates	Fats	Vegetables	Fruit
-Protein Powder -Tofu (can sub tempeh/ seitan)	-Kidney Beans -Black Beans -Mung Beans -Soy Beans -Lentils -Brown Rice -Gluten-free Oats -Flours from above sources -Sweet Potatoes -Yams	-Peanuts -Almonds -Cashews -Nut Butters from above sources -Avocados -Coconut Oil* -Olive Oil* *extra virgin	Kale Spinach Broccoli Lettuce Carrots Cauliflower Onions Peppers	Berries Bananas Apples Pineapple Peaches Mangoes Tomatoes

Stir-Fries
Minimalist Tofu Stir-Fry
Makes 2 servings ~20 minutes, 12 minute/serving w/ reheat

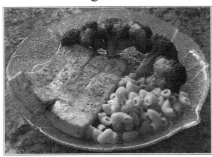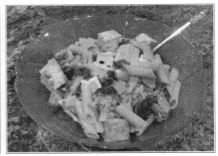

-1 block tofu (400 cal 40g protein) … seasoned with garlic powder, black pepper, etc – can sub tempeh or seitan for tofu
-1 tbsp extra virgin olive oil for pan 120cal 14g fat
-brown rice pasta or other gluten-free pasta ~200cal 41g carb 4g protein
-generous amount of broccoli
-if time, ½ a white onion
per serving: ~380 cal 25g protein ½ serving fat 100cal worth of pasta

1. Large Pan: ~1bsp Olive Oil / Cube a block of tofu. Cover under medium to high heat (your call). Add spices (I use garlic and black pepper).

2. Fire up a small pot of water (enough water for ~200 cals-worth of brown rice pasta or other gluten-free pasta). Bring to a boil.

3. After ~5-7 minutes, "flip" cubes to cook another side. At this point, I add broccoli, onion (opt.), and any other veggies I prefer. I "steam" the broccoli on top of the tofu to avoid charring it. The onions can hit the pan directly if you prefer. Cook for ~5 more minutes, then mix everything and either cook for a few more minutes, or let sit.

4. Once water in pot is boiled, add ~200calories-worth of brown rice pasta or other gluten-free pasta. To estimate this: multiply calories per serving by # of servings, then divide this total number by 200 to find portion size (e.g., 150 x 8 = 1200/200 = 6 | 200cal = 1/6 of box).

If you want a more exact measurement, use a scale to find out how many grams of pasta equals 200 calories (and how this equates to 1 cup dry, ½ cup dry, etc). This only has to be done once, assuming you purchase the same type of pasta over and over again.

5. When pasta finishes, drain and add to stir fry (stir fry will be done by now, turn off heat). Mix the pasta in.

Italian-style Tofu Stir-Fry
Makes 2-3 servings | 20-25minutes

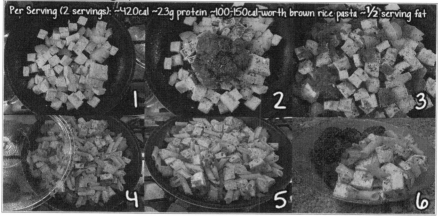

Per Serving (2 servings): ~420cal ~23g protein ~100-150cal worth brown rice pasta ~½ serving fat

1 Block Tofu (can sub tempeh, seitan, etc if you choose) | 1 tbsp Extra Virgin Olive Oil | ~200-300cal worth brown rice pasta or other gluten-free pasta | ½ white onion | 1 small can crushed tomatoes (~14.5oz 3.5servings 30 cal/serv) | garlic, black pepper, basil
Per Serving (2 servings): ~420cal ~23g protein 100-150 cal carbs ~1/2 serving of fat

1. -Add to large pan: 1tbsp EVOO | cubed tofu | season tofu with garlic powder and black pepper - Turn on stove to med-high heat and cover. Also, start heating a separate small pot

-While cooking initial ingredients, slice up a white onion and add to stir fry. Mix in and cover for ~5 minutes.

-After that ~5 minutes flip and stir ingredients to avoid burning / evenly cook ingredients. Cover for ~4 minutes.

2. After that ~4minutes, add in canned crushed tomatoes (no need to drain.. opt.). Before mixing in, season crushed tomatoes with garlic powder and a generous amount of basil. Black pepper opt.

3. Mix in crushed tomatoes, flip and cover for ~5minutes. -Around this time, the water should be at least close to boiling. Add ~200-300 cals worth of brown rice pasta or other gluten-free pasta (penne, elbows, ziti, etc) to pot of water and boil (no need to cover). Guesstimate serving size using box nutrition facts: cals x servings = total cals, then picture what 200-300cals looks like in comparison to that total number! Same concept as prior stir-fry.

-Over next 5-7 minutes, continue to monitor and flip/stir the stir fry and pot of noodles. Test the noodles until desired tenderness.

4. Drain the pot of water/pasta in a strainer and mix pasta into stir fry.

-Stir fry is technically ready, or you can cook the final mixture for a few more minutes if desired. Serve with a side of greens (broccoli).

Thai-style Tofu Stir-Fry (pg. 52)
Makes 3-4 servings | ~ 30 minutes

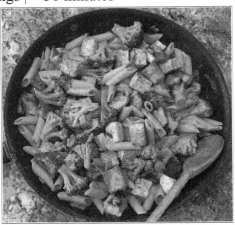

-1 Package Tofu (~400 calories, ~40g protein) ... seasoned with Garlic Powder/Black Pepper (can sub tempeh or seitan for tofu)
-1 tbsp Extra Virgin Olive Oil (~120 calories, 1 serving of fat)

-1 can Thai Coconut Milk (**700 Calories, 5 servings of fat,** ~5g protein)
-1.5 tbsp Red or Green Curry Paste (~23 calories)
-Decent amount of Broccoli (~50+ calories, ~5g protein)
-1 tsp agave (20 calories, ~5g of sugar) – *optional and unnecessary*
-300 calories worth of gluten-free pasta or long-grain rice (~1.5-2 servings worth of carbs, 8g protein)
-Basil (for sauce)
Per Serving (3 servings): ~533 calories, 19g protein, 2 servings of fat, ~½ serving of carbs, tiny amount of sugar (opt., unnecessary)

1. Large Pan: Fry (cubed) tofu in olive oil with garlic powder and black pepper. Flip a few times to evenly cook. Mix in broccoli after ~a flip or two of tofu. Keep broccoli on top of tofu to avoid charring.

2. Small Pan: Mix canned Thai Coconut Milk, Curry Paste, Agave (opt.), and Basil (opt.) → Bring to a boil and then simmer on med-low heat until thickens (this takes at least 10-15 minutes). Stir often.

3. Small to Medium Pot: Boil water, cook pasta or rice until tender/absorbed. Drain and either mix in with stir fry, or keep plain and pour completed stir fry on-top (on each plate).

4. Before the latter part of step 3, combine the sauce from the small pan into everything (tofu & broccoli) that is in the large pan. Stir and cook on low for a few minutes (if need be).

Note: you can also add an onion to this recipe, as well as other vegetables. Do your thing!

This meal is not ideal for cutting. It is a bit too high in fat and calories per serving. If eaten during a cut, eat ¼ of the stir-fry as your portion (~400cals).

Wraps
Making The Actual Wraps

My go-to "bread replacement" is wraps. I make dough from all-purpose gluten free flour, water, and extra virgin olive oil.

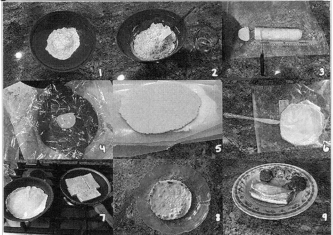

1. Pour some flour into a bowl. Then add a tiny amount of olive oil (a tsp to a tbsp depending on the amount of flour). Slowly add water, little by little.

The key to making dough is the ratio of dry to wet. Too much water creates a "batter-like" consistency-we want dough that we can handle!

2. Mix the ingredients with a spoon/spatula, etc before attempting to knead with your hands. If the product is too moist and sticking to your hands, slowly add flour. If the product is too dry and "crumbly" to create a shape, slowly add a tiny amount of water.

3. When you get the right consistency, form a spherical-like shape and either flatten with a tortilla press (I line the press with plastic bags to prevent sticking), or simply create the wrap-like shape with your hands and fingertips.

I recommend batch cooking ~20+ at a time and storing in the freezer (can use wax paper in between each). To cook, "fry" in a tiny amount of olive oil (~1 tsp) in a small pan. Cook each side for a few minutes (or until desired crispiness).

Basic Tofu Wrap
Follow the instructions in the stir-fry section to fry up the tofu. Instead of cubing the tofu, slice the block into 6 even rectangular sections (while the block lays flat with the largest surface area portions on the top and bottom).

One serving contains ½ of the portion of tofu (3 slices) and 1 wrap. I place 2 of the rectangular pieces of tofu inside the wrap, and eat one on the side, usually with some broccoli. I use the rest of the tofu to make another wrap to eat in a few hours. (Can bring both to work)
Per Serving (w/ broccoli): ~360cals 25g protein 120cals of carbs

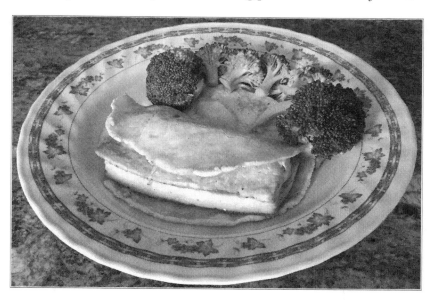

Smoothies

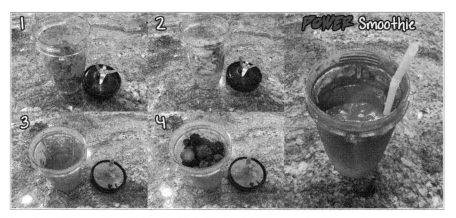

Note: these pictures are intended for the EBOOK. It is difficult to see them in print!

Berry-based Smoothie
Plant protein powder, peanut butter, mixed berries, kale or spinach, water and/or non-dairy milk (cashew milk, almond milk, etc … unsweetened).

1. Add kale or spinach to a smoothie cup (fresh or frozen). If you are concerned about taste, add just a small amount for your first time. Increase the amount little by little each time you make one. Take my word for it: these taste great even with a very large amount of greens!

2. Add 1 scoop of protein powder (~120cals 20+g protein), 2 TBSP of Peanut Butter (can use any nut butter), and fill the cup ~half way with water and/or almond or cashew milk (can sub in any unsweetened, low calorie, non-dairy milk).

3. Blend this initial concoction before adding fruit. This allows the greens to liquefy instead of a "chopped up" result when combined with too many ingredients. This pre-blend is also easier on the blender.

4. Add frozen mixed berries to the initial blend. I prioritize strawberries, then add any combination of: blueberries, blackberries, and/or raspberries (as much as I can fit or desire). You can use fresh fruit, however frozen fruit creates a milkshake-type consistency and temperature. It tastes far, far, better with frozen fruit. You may need to add a tad bit more water/non-dairy milk to these final spins.

Calories: ~375-400 / Protein: ~30g+ / Carb: 20-30g / Fat: ~17g (The carbs are all from fruit, greens, and the peanut butter. These numbers can vary depending on the amount of fruit, greens, and the type of protein powder. If bulking, feel free to add more peanut butter and potentially protein powder. Oats are an option here as well.)

Tropical-based Smoothie
Same as the smoothie above, except: strawberries as the base + peaches, mangoes, pineapple, etc.

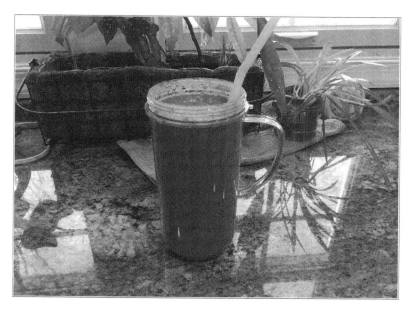

Oatmeals
Blueberry Oatmeal (w/ protein drink & broccoli on the side)
1. Bring 1 cup of water to a boil. Add 1/2 cup of quick cooking gluten-free oats. Cook for a few minutes until desired consistency. (Can microwave instead if no access to stove.) Mix in rinsed, raw blueberries. (~a handful)

2. Rinsed raw broccoli on side. (Can use any green-kale, spinach, etc). Try to get this green in if possible!

3. 1 scoop protein powder mixed with ice water. The colder the better. (Tastes better cold.)
Calories: ~375 / Protein: 31g / Carb: 53g / Fat: 4.5g
(32g carb from oats ... can add more oats if bulking)

Banana Cinnamon Peanut Butter Oatmeal
Cook your oats plain (#1 above) → Slice a banana and place on top of oats → sprinkle cinnamon on top of banana → drip a small amount of natural peanut butter on top of each banana piece (or a swirl)→ do not mix! take spoonfuls from the bottom to create a layer of oats, banana, cinnamon, and pb! (Go easy on the PB, it's caloric. Use ½ to 1 tbsp tops.)

Compared to the blueberry oatmeal above, this version will be 50-100 more calories—another ¼ to ½ serving of fat (from the peanut butter). This is more of a bulk/maintenance meal. If eating during a cut, either eliminate the peanut butter, or use just under ½ cup of oats and only ¼ tbsp of peanut butter.

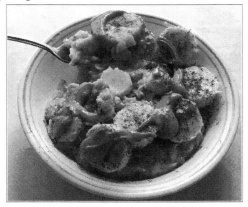

Index

About The Author

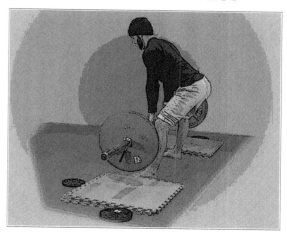

M.G. Green is the pen name of an author that has over a decade of experience in the fitness industry. He has worked with everyone from "weekend warriors" to Division-1 athletes. He specializes in the areas of corrective exercise, strength and conditioning, and nutrition.

After experimenting with a multitude of diets, M.G. Green eventually converted to a Vegan lifestyle. His goal was to create a healthy diet on the basis of morality and efficiency, without sacrificing taste and effectiveness. The result: *Plant Based Diet Manual: Proven Strategies To Lose Weight & Gain Muscle On A Plant Based Diet.*

For recipes, diet tips, fitness tips, and "before and after" photos, check out his Instagram page:
https://www.instagram.com/fiveminutediet/

If you enjoyed this book, I would greatly appreciate it if you could leave a review on Amazon.com! This ultimately helps me write more books in related genres.

Thank you for reading!

Printed in Great Britain
by Amazon